# MAKE A DIFFERENCE WITH MENTAL HEALTH ACTIVISM

*No Activism Degree Required—Use Your Unique Skills to Change the World*

TERRI L. LYON

TRISH LOCKARD

Based on the *What's On Your Sign?* 5-Step Activism Path

Make a Difference with Mental Health Activism
No activism degree required—use your unique skills to change the world
Written by Terri L. Lyon and Trish Lockard
 Published in the United States by Life At The Intersection Books, Maryville, Tennessee. For information contact:
admin@lifeattheintersection.com https://lifeattheintersection.com

Cataloging Information
Names: Lyon, Terri, author and Lockard, Trish, author
Title: Make a Difference with Mental Health Activism
No activism degree required—use your unique skills to change the world
Terri L. Lyon and Trish Lockard
Description: First Edition / Tennessee: Life At The Intersection Books, 2021 / Includes bibliographical references and index.
Paperback ISBN: 978-0-9980324-6-7
Social Science-Volunteer Work
Medical-Health Policy
Book cover design: bittereva
Editor: Trish Lockard/Strike The Write Tone
Author photos: Mark Empey Photography
First Edition: September 2021
Printed in the United States of America
10 9 8 7 6 5 4 3 2 1

# DEDICATION

*I dedicate this book to all who came before me.*

*—Terri Lyon*

*To all the mothers, fathers, siblings, and spouses I have worked with through the National Alliance on Mental Illness, NAMI, I dedicate this book to you for the never-wavering care and resilience you show for your loved ones.*

*—Trish Lockard*

# ADVANCE PRAISE FOR *MAKE A DIFFERENCE WITH MENTAL HEALTH ACTIVISM*

**After 30 years in psychiatry, I had no idea how to do activism. After reading Lyon's and Lockard's *Make a Difference with Mental Health Activism*, I now know just what to do and where to find much more information. I urge anyone who wants to do even the smallest amount to make a difference for mental health advancement to read this book.**

MARK D. REGO, MD, ASSISTANT CLINICAL PROFESSOR OF PSYCHIATRY, YALE SCHOOL OF MEDICINE AND AUTHOR OF *FRONTAL FATIGUE: THE IMPACT OF MODERN LIFE AND TECHNOLOGY ON MENTAL ILLNESS*

***Make a Difference with Mental Health Activism* is a book every activist needs, whether you've been one for years or are just thinking about becoming one. It covers everything from bringing out your inner activist to learning how to use your own passions and skills to make your voice heard. Full of ideas, examples, and personal stories, this book is a wonderful guide down the path to activism.**

VINCENT M. WALES

AWARD-WINNING NOVELIST, FREETHOUGHT ACTIVIST, FORMER MENTAL HEALTH PODCASTER & SUICIDE PREVENTION COUNSELOR

# About the Activism Path Books

Each book based on the *Activism Path* focuses on a specific topic. The books walk you along a path to identify what you are passionate about, what you're angry about, what you're good at, and what you enjoy. Our hope is that you will turn what you learn about yourself into action.

The focus of this book is *mental health.* Woven throughout your journey along the path are profiles of some of this country's most passionate mental health activists. Some might be familiar to you; others will be a revelation.

These activists make a difference as authors, crafters, podcasters, artists, and coalition builders—folks who are tapping into their talents to make change happen. Learn what drives their passion for mental health activism and reform. It is our hope that their stories will inspire you and get your own creative activism juices flowing.

By journey's end, you will be empowered to use your skills, talents, and experience to act on behalf of those with mental health disorders, their families, and society as a whole.

What will you do? Are you a writer? Business manager? Crafter? Musician? Bookkeeper? Painter? Social media whiz? Quilter? Comedian? Website designer? A loving parent, spouse, or friend?

We will lead you, with all you have to offer, to an ideal activism opportunity.

Become an effective activist for those with mental health disorders and for families that care for them.

For yourself. For your loved ones. For your community.

The time for change is now.

# The Mental Health Activism Companion Website

*Make a Difference with Mental Health Activism* has a Mental Health Activism Companion Website. You can access notes, downloadable worksheets, links, and additional resources, which will help you get the most from the book.

The website is at:

https://lifeattheintersection.com/mental-health-activism-companion/

# Contents

Foreword ........ 1

Preface ........ 5

Who Is This Book For? ........ 6

You're Crazy! ........ 7

"I can't afford my meds; We can't find a therapist." ........ 8

Mental Health Emerges from the Closet ........ 9

The Roots of Mental Health Activism ........ 11

Mental Health Activism Today—It's Your Turn ........ 12

Introduction ........ 13

*Your Path to Change the World for Those with Mental Illness*

The Activism Path ........ 13

Why Follow the Activism Path? ........ 16

What's Next? ........ 17

Chapter 1 ........ 19

*Your Passion—Mental Health*

Activist in Action: Christinea Beane ........ 20

Creating a Life Vision ........ 23

Want to Learn More? ........ 26

What's Next? ........ 27

Chapter 2 ........ 29

*Inventory Your Gifts*

Activist in Action: Christina Wolfgram ........ 29

Your Gifts ........ 32

Clarify Your Motivation ........ 34

Want to Learn More? ........ 36

What's Next? ........ 38

Chapter 3 .......... 39
*Mental Health Activism Techniques*
Activist in Action: Karyl Chastain Beal .......... 39
Traditional Approaches to Mental Health Activism .......... 42
Creative Approaches to Mental Health Activism .......... 47
Summary .......... 58
The Right Activism Method for You .......... 58
Want to Learn More? .......... 59
What's Next? .......... 60
Chapter 4 .......... 61
*Activism That Makes an Impact*
Activist in Action: Miana Bryant .......... 62
Your Activism Opportunities .......... 64
Brainstorm Your Options .......... 65
Narrow Your Options with a Focus on Impact .......... 67
Want to Learn More? .......... 69
What's Next? .......... 70
Chapter 5 .......... 71
*Your Action Plan to Stay Motivated*
Activist in Action: Gabe Howard .......... 71
Your Action Plan .......... 74
Create Your Action Plan .......... 74
Want to Learn More? .......... 77
What's Next? .......... 78
Conclusion .......... 79
*You Can Be a Mental Health Activist*
What You Learned from the Activism Path .......... 79
Tips from the Activists in Action .......... 80
Be There for Others .......... 86

Afterword .......... 87
Mental Health Resources .......... 91
Helplines .......... 91
Organizations .......... 91
Books .......... 92
Podcasts .......... 93
Acknowledgments .......... 95
Also Available .......... 97
About the Authors .......... 99
*Trish Lockard* .......... *99*
*Terri Lyon* .......... *101*
Index .......... 103
Notes .......... 107

# FOREWORD

**Mental illness is a cruel disease.**

—PETE EARLEY, AUTHOR OF CRAZY: A FATHER'S SEARCH THROUGH AMERICA'S MENTAL HEALTH MADNESS

Our mental health care system is a mess. It is difficult to get meaningful care unless you become so sick that you act out and then, there is a higher probability that you will be arrested and punished, rather than being helped. This is wrong. The most effective way for us to push for reforms and improve our mental health system is by exposing barriers to care, and the most effective way to accomplish that is by putting human faces on the problems. The community and our elected leaders must realize that mental illnesses impact millions of Americans.

NAMI and the National Institute of Mental Health claim that as many as one in four Americans will experience some type of mental illness during their lifetimes. [Editor's note: During the COVID-19 pandemic, that statistic jumped to one in three.] Telling our stories humanizes the illness. People with mental illnesses are not simply statistics. They are our parents, our brothers and sisters, our children, and our neighbors. Not speaking out encourages stigma.

There should be no shame in having a mental illness, only shame in not helping someone who does.

As the father of an adult son with a mental illness, I have an obligation to share our story because doing so helps fight stigma and because what happened to my son exposes the failures in our system. Because my son finally got the help that he needed, our story offers hope to others. [Editor's note: Read more about Pete's son Kevin Earley in this book's Acknowledgments.]

After my personal experiences, I want people to know that my son's breakdown and the six years that we went through together—the arrests, the hospitalizations, the arguments—helped all of us to grow. It opened our hearts and gave both my son and me a purpose in life. Because my son finally got the help that he needed, he was able to become a full-time, peer-to-peer specialist and obtained a master's degree in social work. His success offers hope to others that someone they love also cannot only survive a mental illness but thrive.

I would encourage those reading *Make a Difference with Mental Health Activism* to get involved in the campaign to improve mental health services.

Join NAMI, Mental Health America, or the Treatment Advocacy Center. If you get involved, you will not only help others, but your life will be enriched too, because you will have a purpose greater than yourself. There is so much need. Answer the call.

Pete Earley

*Pete Earley has had an illustrious career. After a fourteen-year stint in journalism, including six years at* The Washington Post, *Pete became a full-time author with a commitment to expose the stories that entertain and surprise. He later began writing novels, as he says, for fun, but he now has penned twenty-one books including four* New York Times *bestsellers, such as* The Hot House.[1]

*Another of his bestsellers is his most personal and heart-wrenching, the 2007 Pulitzer Prize finalist* Crazy: A Father's Search Through America's Mental Health Madness.[2] *When Pete's life was turned upside down by the events recounted in that book,* he joined the National Alliance on Mental Illness[3] *(NAMI) to advocate publicly for strong mental health reform.*

# Preface

**What mental health needs is more sunlight, more candor, and more unashamed conversation.**

—GLENN CLOSE, ACTOR AND ACTIVIST

Throughout history, the symptoms of mental illness have caused fear, superstition, and condemnation. Some would say that, even now in the twenty-first century, we still have a long way to go. These statistics bear out the impact of mental illness:

- ✓ Found in 45% of the homeless (30% of these have serious mental illness, such as schizophrenia)
- ✓ Found in 56% of state prisoners, 45% of federal prisoners, and 64% of jail inmates
- ✓ Directly linked to illicit drug use and alcohol and prescription medication misuse
- ✓ Costs the nation at least $193 billion annually in lost earnings
- ✓ Found in 95% of youth who die by suicide
- ✓ Found in 41% of war veterans
- ✓ Forces 8.4 million Americans to provide daily in-home care for a loved one

Mental health disorders are at the core of the worst of our country's societal and economic problems.

## Who Is This Book For?

*Make a Difference with Mental Health Activism* is for you if:

- ✓ You are the 1 in 6 children and teens (7.7 million) in the United States with a mental health diagnosis who lives this reality every day (9.7% or 2.3 million youth aged 12-17 have severe major depression.)
- ✓ You are the 1 in 5 adults (51.5 million) in the United States with a mental health diagnosis, the lived experience, who knows the impact all too well. (According to the CDC, this number doubled to 2 in 5 by early 2021.)
- ✓ You are the 1 in 8.4 million caregivers of someone with a diagnosis.
- ✓ You are a friend, neighbor, or coworker of someone with mental illness.
- ✓ You are someone who has compassion for another human being who, through no fault of their own, does not always have control over their thoughts, feelings, and behavior.

## You're Crazy!

If you have a mental health diagnosis—the lived experience, as it's called—have you ever been called *crazy*? It hurts, doesn't it? Have you ever called someone else crazy or used other hurtful language?

*"Jesse's just psycho."*

*"That guy acted like a complete nutjob."*

*"Lauren is a total schizo!"*

Begin to pay attention to how often you hear people refer to others as *crazy, nuts, insane, wacky, psycho, loony, nutjob,* etc. We have become numb to thoughtless social vernacular that is hurtful to people with a mental health diagnosis and those who love them.

Name-calling is one form of *stigma*. So, what is stigma?

*Stigma is when someone views you in a negative way because you have a distinguishing characteristic or personal trait that's thought to be, or actually is, a disadvantage (a negative stereotype).*

*—Mayo Clinic, 2017*

Stigma is the number one reason people with mental illness are laughed at, misunderstood, bullied, and discriminated against. People who do not seek treatment for their mental illness cite stigma as the primary reason.

Mental health activism must be employed to end the shame attached to mental illness.

## "I can't afford my meds; We can't find a therapist."

This book's cowriter Trish Lockard has taught NAMI's flagship program Family-to-Family many times. She has also facilitated and participated in many NAMI family support group meetings. The most common topic of conversation—and the one that brings with it the most anger—is the inaccessibility of affordable medications, treatment facilities, and therapists/counselors. Even families with what would be considered good health insurance often cannot afford or find help for their loved ones. Why is this? It has to do with the way mental health has been viewed by the medical community throughout history and how insurance companies have discriminated against behavioral health—and gotten away with it.

Organizations like NAMI and Mental Health America have been loud voices on behalf of this discrimination for decades. And those loud voices eventually paid off. According to MHA:

*Lack of understanding regarding mental health and deep-rooted stigma help explain why it is still so common for health plans to place greater restrictions on treating behavioral health disorders than on other illnesses. While enlightened business leaders in some industries and communities have voluntarily provided parity protection for their workforces, voluntary measures are not an answer to the widespread discrimination facing most insured Americans. Thus, Mental Health America supports insurance-parity legislation.*[4]

As defined by the Substance Abuse and Mental Health Services Administration (SAMHSA), parity means *the state or condition of being equal (in status).* Lack of parity in mental health services creates heartache and puts those with the lived experience and their families in peril. Thanks in large part to the 2008 Mental Health Parity and Addiction Equity Act (MHPAEA or "parity act"), numerous changes to how insurance companies would cover mental and behavioral health condition expenses improved dramatically.

However, even with the passage of MHPAEA, anyone with an addiction or mental health diagnosis knows that the playing field is still far from level.

We must continue to fight for health care equality for those with addiction and mental illness. Mental health is health!

## Mental Health Emerges from the Closet

The year 2020 saw a dramatic rise in discussions about mental health disorders. Global news headlines and television broadcasts shone a spotlight on the increase in diagnoses of anxiety and depression as a direct result of the COVID-19 pandemic.

In fact, experts called this increase the *underlying crisis* of the pandemic. While COVID-19 cases spiked around the country in 2020, more than one third of Americans reported related symptoms of anxiety and depression. According to Dr. James O'Dea, vice president of operations for the Hartford HealthCare Behavioral Health Network,

*The spread of COVID-19 leaves people feeling out of control, which is uncomfortable and unnerving. We're driven to protect ourselves and loved ones from perceived threats and the uncertainty surrounding this situation escalates fears.*

According to 2020 Census Bureau statistics, 24% of 42,000 respondents reported significant symptoms of major depressive disorder and 30% reported symptoms of generalized anxiety disorder, which were, in some cases, *double* those reported in 2014.

This book's co-author Trish Lockard wrote an article about this rise in first-time mental health diagnoses for the website Life At The Intersection: "Think the Pandemic Was Hard? Consider the Impact on Those with Mental Illness."[5]

For the last several years, a wide range of celebrities have used their high-profile public platforms to speak openly about their own struggles with mental health disorders. England's Prince Harry, singer/actor Demi Lovato, rapper Kendrick Lamar, even superhero actors Chris Evans and Ryan Reynolds have shared stories about the shame and trauma they felt and the exhaustion of hiding their mental illness symptoms for years.

And in the sports world, tennis champ Naomi Osaka and gymnast Simone Biles retreated from competition when mental health challenges got the best of them during huge athletic events. In an interview with NBC's Lester Holt, Olympic swimming legend Michael Phelps, who openly struggled with depression during his swimming career, publicly congratulated both women on their bravery and wished such high-profile examples of mental health challenges will result in worldwide conversation and understanding. Let's hope Michael is right![6]

## The Roots of Mental Health Activism

**Every evil has its good, and every ill an antidote.**

—DOROTHEA DIX

Activism on behalf of those with mental health disorders is not a twenty-first-century movement.

In the 1840s, Dorothea Dix was a teacher, lobbyist, and superintendent of nurses during the Civil War. An outspoken, no-nonsense woman, Dix was appalled by the conditions in which those diagnosed with mental illnesses were confined. She became a social reformer and author dedicated to changing conditions for people who could not help themselves, a crusader for the mentally ill and the imprisoned.

Through her tireless work over four decades, Dix instituted changes in the treatment and care of the mentally ill and improved prison conditions. She successfully persuaded the US government to fund the building of psychiatric hospitals. Between 1843 and 1880, she helped to establish thirty-two new mental hospitals across the US—including in New York, Indiana, Illinois, Rhode Island, and Tennessee—and she aided in improving the care of many more.

Today, the results of her efforts can still be seen throughout the United States, Canada, and many European countries.

## Mental Health Activism Today—It's Your Turn

Whether you have a diagnosis or are a family member, caregiver, or friend of someone who does, those with mental health disorders are a chronically underrepresented and misunderstood population. They face shortages of mental health workers, lack of research capacity, stigma, and the segregation of mental health services from other physical and medical health services.

Activism could be the difference between continued stigma, lack of parity, and shame of those with mental health disorders and advanced awareness, increased services, and emotional support.

**Mental illness is nothing to be ashamed of, but stigma and bias shame us all.**

—BILL CLINTON, FORMER PRESIDENT

The time for change is now.

# INTRODUCTION

## YOUR PATH TO CHANGE THE WORLD FOR THOSE WITH MENTAL ILLNESS

**A journey of a thousand miles begins with a single step.**

—LAO-TZU, CHINESE PHILOSOPHER

How wonderful that you want to make a difference for those with mental illness and their caregivers and loved ones. Let us help you find the best way to do this.

What is *activism*? Activism is any action meant to influence others to support your cause. It refers to a behavioral chance, whereas *advocacy*, which is also vitally important to change, involves eliciting a change to public policy.

### The Activism Path

Dr. Terri Lyon's 2018 ground-breaking book *What's On Your Sign? How to focus your passion and change the world*[7] introduced new activists to the 5-step Activism Path, a road map to better recognize your talents and experiences and passions. The 5-step path helps you:

1. find your passions,
2. identify your gifts,

3. craft your ideal opportunities,
4. monitor your success, and
5. stay motivated.

With *Make a Difference with Mental Health Activism*, you will travel that same Activism Path. Each chapter does not have the same level of detail presented in *What's On Your Sign*? but provides a comprehensive overview of the process, more than enough to get you going. It is a great jumping-off point for both new and experienced activists. Here is a preview of your journey on the Activism Path.

## Step 1: Focus Your Passion

Since you already know your number one activism passion—mental health—in step 1 you focus your passion. Don't get overwhelmed trying to solve every problem. Clarify your image of the ideal life and ideal world and find the cause that means the most to you. Focus on this and become more effective. If you choose the cause closest to your heart, you stay motivated.

And it is not just your passion for a cause, although that is a goal. It is about the way you want to live your life. Create a life vision where you picture how you are living your life and your values. Once you understand that, you can imagine how your mental health activism fits into the picture. How much time can you spend on it while still being a partner, parent, employee?

Can you see how this might help you in many ways in your life? For activism, it means more impact. Activists who focus their efforts rather than taking a scattershot approach are more effective.

## Step 2: Clarify Your Unique Skills

With your primary passion decided, this step on the Activism Path is to inventory the gifts—skills, knowledge, and motivation—you will bring to this activism work. This step requires self-reflection and insight. Why?

Because if you use the skills and knowledge you already possess, you'll be more effective. And if you're more effective, you'll be more motivated and engaged.

Everyone has something they do well, talents that come naturally to you or skills you have acquired. When you are tuned into your highest-level talents and skills, you can match them to your activism work.

## Step 3: Do Activism You Love

Consider your options for various activism methods. By recognizing your gifts, you can find a method that will light your fire.

For example, some people like to work in a team, while others prefer working alone. Which are you?

Suppose the thought of speaking with or writing to your elected officials gives you anxiety. In that case, those aren't the right activism methods for you. On the other hand, if you love to write, start cranking out letters to your representatives. Write articles for a local paper or magazine. Get blogging!

### Step 4: Make a Difference

We're all busy. The time you spend on activism is precious, so make it count. When you have matched your gifts and method to your passion, make sure the work you choose makes a real difference to a person, a group, or an organization.

In this step, you learn ways to measure the potential impact of your activism choices, so you can pick the one with the most bang.

### Step 5: See Change Happen

The last step on the Activism Path is to change the world! Or, at least, as much of it as you can reasonably influence.

Ready yourself by setting goals that will motivate you and celebrate your progress, while keeping you focused on achieving the best results from your work.

And while you are working for the greater good, recognize signs of stress. Beware of burnout!

Sometimes activism is hard, and it is vital to take care of yourself. By identifying when you are stressed and managing it before it overwhelms you, you'll be able to make change happen for a longer time. Successful activists make sure their work motivates them because the work can be challenging at times.

## Why Follow the Activism Path?

Before you get started in your mental health activism, take time to reflect. Why is being thoughtful before you begin your activism important? You want to enjoy your activism, make real change happen, and stay motivated.

How?

Follow the Activism Path to ensure deeper engagement and more impact.

When new activists leap in without preparation, they tend to drop out. Only 2% of activists stay for the long-term. We need every mental health activist motivated and engaged.

The Activism Path activities cannot be completed in a day. Instead, the best results come from reflection on your life and your cause. Being thoughtful from the get-go will pay off for you and for those you most desire to help.

Change must come from the ground up. Individuals. Families. Places of work. Houses of worship. In fact, individual efforts grow and spread to ever-higher tiers of power and authority. Grassroots activism breaks down obstacles and puts mental wellness and well-being for all within our reach.

Let's get started.

## What's Next?

In Chapter 1, you will learn how to focus your mental health passion.

In Chapter 2, you will examine the skills, knowledge, and motivation you bring to activism.

Chapter 3 is chock-full of mental health activism techniques, so you can find the one that's perfect for you.

In Chapter 4, you will look at the ways you can make the most impact.

Finally, in Chapter 5, you'll examine how to put your activism into action, evaluate how you're doing, and stay motivated.

Let's start with an example of an activist who made a lovely match between her passion and gifts.

# CHAPTER 1

## YOUR PASSION—MENTAL HEALTH

**Give me six hours to chop down a tree and I will spend the first four sharpening the axe.**

—ABRAHAM LINCOLN

It's time to begin your journey along the Activism Path. When you have many causes you want to support, it's hard to choose one and focus only on it. Since you are reading this book, we know you have a passion for mental health issues and improving the treatments, services, and social conditions for those in need. So, that's one step down, four to go.

But wait! Even though you have found your passion, don't skip this chapter.

So many aspects of mental health care need to be changed; you might find it hard to choose the one that's perfect for you. This chapter will guide you to focus on your *specific* passion within this issue.

### Why Focus Your Passion?

Read the Abraham Lincoln quote at the beginning of the chapter. He knows that if he prepares his axe well, chopping down the tree will be much easier. Similarly, you will be most effective making a difference in mental health if you first focus your passion.

Even focusing on mental health, you could still find yourself spread thin—raising funds, facilitating a support group, writing letters to the editor, and teaching classes. You get the picture.

Instead, find a way to combine your passion with your talents and skills and a method that most motivates you. The way Christinea Beane has.

## Activist in Action: Christinea Beane

*Christinea Beane is a jewelry-maker extraordinaire. Her Makes Cents Jewelry*[8] *started with a care package to a total stranger and the intention to stimulate conversation and generate awareness for mental illness. Christinea sees the penny as a metaphor for everything in life (hence, her business name), using art as a form of expression, and coming closer to see how things work beneath the surface. She created a jewelry line that incorporates a penny, guitar strings, and gears in every piece.*

*Christinea has talked openly about her own struggle with depression and suicidal ideations. She has lost dear ones to suicide.*

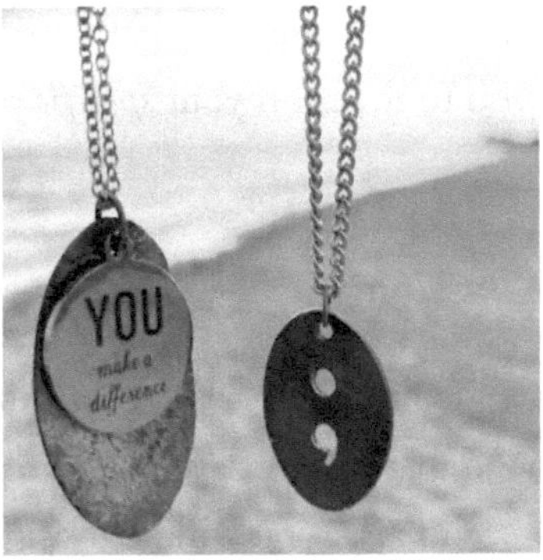

Why is it important for me to advocate on behalf of mental health? To create a sense of belonging. To help find support and community. To bring hope and support to those who feel as though they are losing their battle. To remind people they are not alone. I need support, hope, and community for myself and I hope to bring these to others who need them too.

When I receive a request for a custom piece, I ask questions to understand the person's story. Not one of our stories is better or worse than another and not one version is harder than the next. It's just hard. Those stories, your story, became the inspiration for Makes Cents Jewelry and every piece is painstakingly created to create safe places to share your story.

Through Makes Cents Jewelry, I encourage open conversation and normalize mental health issues. When I talk about the items I incorporate into my pieces and why it's important to me, I work to fight stigma and provide a safe place for those like me to openly reflect on their illnesses and challenges.

I suppose I could measure my success by looking at my sales and income. But I know it's about far more than that. The measurement of how vital my work is comes from the conversations I have and the feedback I receive. There is a ripple effect that I will never be able to comprehend.

I fought against the idea of medication management for the longest time. I was dishonest with myself for many years, thus I was dishonest with the people who could help. When I really wanted to crawl out from beneath the negative thoughts, I had to be honest and accept that I could not do it alone. When I looked at the health of my brain in the same way as the health of my body, I used the same language—*I am sick*. When I think about my habits when I am physically sick, I began to notice the similarities to when I am mentally sick. Those similarities created unhealthy habits, fostered unhealthy relationships, and stalled the healing process.

I don't feel I have chosen to be a mental health advocate. I don't think I really had any choice—it is the right thing for me to do. When I talk with folks, I rely on facts not feelings. What worked for me might not work for others. I ask questions and build trust by listening without judgment. Nothing says "I am listening" like silence.

♦ ♦ ♦

Christinea's story reminds us that we can make our passion a guiding light. In fact, she gave up her job to focus on her jewelry because she is passionate about listening to people's stories.

She donates a portion of her profits to the national organization To Write Love On Her Arms,[9] which also focuses on listening to and sharing people's stories.

## Finding Your Specific Passion

A passion for mental health might hit you in the face when you are not expecting it. Perhaps your diagnosis, or the diagnosis of a loved one, sets you on the path. You might be like Christinea in finding your passion in this way.

But sometimes, your specific passion is buried deep within the trappings of your life.

## Creating a Life Vision

Your roles, personal values, and past life experiences paint a picture of your passions.

One way to clarify your passions—and we mean in all areas of your life, not just activism—is to create your life vision. By drawing yourself from the present into the future, you imagine your ideal life.

Here is an example.

Former teacher and amateur community theater actor Tami is passionate about ending stigma toward kids with a diagnosis. Using her background in theater, she wrote and produced a play for elementary schools, highlighting the impact of stigma. The audiences' responses have been heartwarming. She wakes up every day excited about her activism. Tami spent time reflecting on her roles, values, and wishes and created a life vision that worked perfectly for her. Her reflection brought her to these statements about herself:

*I incorporate compassion in my roles of mother, spouse, friend, client, and athlete. My values include:*

*I support my family and the people I serve as a caregiver, including my younger sibling with Depressive Disorder.*

*I am mentally and physically healthy.*

*I focus on the experiences of the present moment.*

*I give back to my community.*

*I have fun!*

Using this list as a focal point, she rearranged her priorities. She spent more time with her family. Because she is a caregiver, she identified her activism passion as helping other caregivers with stress awareness and coping strategies. In the end, she switched from theater to teach yoga and meditation to other caregivers. This combination of her passion, skills, and motivation suits her perfectly.

Notice how Tami's life vision includes her values and essential roles. She uses her life vision to guide her life decisions.

Creating a life vision might take time, but it will be a North Star guiding you for the rest of your life. It will keep you focused on the values and roles most important to you. When it comes to activism, it is easy to tell yourself, "I will get to that later." Instead, a life vision makes a place in your life for helping others.

## Focusing on Love

Another way to be specific about your passion is to start with what you love.

Here is an example:

Copywriter Lauren Weiss struggled with her mental health for years, knowing that something was wrong. But she succumbed to the stigma toward mental illness and particularly against using medications for treatment. She finally decided to seek help and was diagnosed with bipolar disorder II and given a prescription.

*My brain felt clear for the first time. I was more creative, more productive, more myself because I wasn't being derailed by mania or depression all the time. It blew my mind that people actually lived a mentally stable life even with a diagnosis.*

She loved her new life and wanted to make sure others didn't allow stigma to stand in the way of getting help. So, she created #WearYourMeds,[10] buttons that look like common psychotropic medications. Her goal is to facilitate conversations about mental illness.

*I'm not a mental health or medical professional. I know that meds are not the answer for everyone, and I would never make any attempt to diagnose or medicate anyone. But my hope is that #WearYourMeds will normalize the mental illness conversation, let people tell their stories, and pay it forward for people who might be struggling to pursue professional help from people who made that journey.*

## Focusing on Anger

Love is an excellent method to help focus on your passion. Another way to focus your passion is to consider what makes you angry or breaks your heart. Tap into that anger.

For example, a teacher who got angry when several of her students acted out took a step back and recognized that they were likely living with various traumatic experiences at home. She asked the school system's counselors to administer the Adverse Childhood Experiences (ACEs) Assessment test. An ACE score is a tally of different types of abuse, neglect, and other adverse childhood experiences. A higher score indicates a higher risk for health problems, including mental health problems, later in life. The teacher channeled her initial anger at the children into a step toward support and help for her students.

### Learning from Your Past

Look back at your life experiences. What life choices have you made? Why did you make them? We all have lessons we've learned that we can use to make better choices in the future.

What are the threads that tie all your life experiences together? Tug the mental health thread a bit and note all the places where your passion for this issue made itself known.

When Ben was young, he loved psychological thrillers and read books like *The Bell Jar*. He used his camcorder in high school to make a film about students who didn't live in a stable home. He became a social worker, hoping to help homeless men and women get off the streets. Ben's mental health thread led him to a career helping the homeless.

## Want to Learn More?

We hope these activist stories have shown you the power of using your passion in a specific way to help those with mental illness.

Take sufficient time for this step on the Activism Path. You will be more motivated and effective in your activism—and you might find your life is enhanced and fruitful in myriad ways.

Below are additional resources for those who want the chance to get more detail about a topic.

If you are ready to move on, go to What's Next?

### Additional Resources

1. Terri Lyon's books *What's On Your Sign?*[11] and *The What's On Your Sign? Workbook*[12] offer a structured approach to finding the perfect activism opportunity for you. One that makes a difference for those you love, doing something you love. Get exercises, worksheets, checklists, and reflective questions to help you identify your passion.
2. Visit Terri's website Life At The Intersection and start with the blog post "How To Create A Vision Of a Joyful Life."[13]
3. The societal effects of mental illness are all around us. For more proof, read Trish Lockard's article on the website Life At The Intersection, "With Mental Illness, You Won't Get a Casserole."[14]

## What's Next?

We hope Christinea's story has shown you the power of using your passion to make a change for those with mental illness. Christinea matched her passion with her artistic gifts and is living her values every day.

If you are specific about your passion, you can do the same.

In the next chapter, you will explore step 2 on the Activism Path: understanding your gifts.

You'll meet another Christina, who uses her gifts in a unique and witty way. What's funny about mental illness? Read on.

# CHAPTER 2

## INVENTORY YOUR GIFTS

**Be a lamp, a lifeboat, a ladder. Help someone's soul heal. Walk out of your house like a shepherd.**

—RUMI

When you imagine mental health activism, you probably don't think of comedy. But Christina Wolfgram, self-described *internet comedian and expert public crier*, uses her gift for comedy in a podcast for women to pursue good mental health. Many mental health podcasts are heavy, like a therapy session. But *Sobcast the Podcast*[15] is different—funny and relatable.

### Activist in Action: Christina Wolfgram

*Christina Wolfgram is a writer and video producer who specializes in comedy for women. A self-described* sit-down comedian, *her videos have been viewed more than 500 million times on Facebook and Instagram. Her hit "When you suck at eyeliner" remains Time Inc.'s highest-viewed video ever at 60 million views. Most recently, Christina entered the wide world of podcasting with* Sobcast the Podcast, *through which she asks listeners to join her on her journey of figuring out what mental health even means.*

*We asked Christina about her journey.*

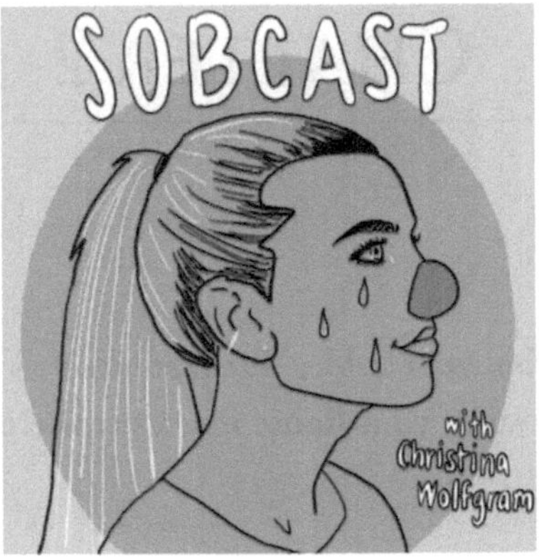


When I was struggling with my depression most (I'm talking, not being able to get out of bed, crying in the bathroom at work, consumed with horrible thoughts), I saw a YouTube video of a comedian that I've followed for years where she talked about taking Lexapro. I couldn't believe that someone I loved and laughed with like that could be dealing with similar struggles to my own. My goal is to be that person for others; I don't get embarrassed talking about mental health, so I'm more than happy to start the conversation for those who don't know where to start.

My goal is to empower others to find what works for them when it comes to mental health. No one has all the answers because no two brains are the same! It's okay to try different methods and it's more than okay to change your routine when you need to. Beyond that, I want to make people laugh. Being a human being is freaking ridiculous.

I do what I do and don't concern myself with stats about viewership or listenership. I've gotten caught up in stats a few times in my life, and I've realized the most vital thing (for me) is to continue making truthful content. When I make comedy videos, I create characters who are pretending they have their sh*t together, when in reality they are struggling to be *normal.* Some of those videos have been shared by huge audiences, and I like to think it's because people relate to that feeling. It's cool to see those viewership numbers go up, but it's even more important to me when I get an email from someone saying they played my podcast for a loved one to start a conversation about their depression.

Three years ago, I was at my lowest point mental health-wise. Seriously, I didn't know I was capable of holding so much sadness and worry in my body. I started taking medication as part of my mental health routine (which also includes therapy, bothering my cat, and moving my body), and I feel like I'm only just noticing how much of an impact that routine has had on my life. How? Because emails don't make me cry anymore!

You don't have to pretend like you have any answers. It can be *so* confusing to be on Instagram, scrolling past hundreds of posts that curtly state that Vitamin D will cure your depression, or that getting enough sleep will cure your depression, or *we're all in this together* and that should cure your depression. Nope! It's different for everyone and there is absolutely *not* a simple solution that will magically transform everyone's lives.

Be kind and listen. Being a part of the conversation is already helping more than you know!

♦ ♦ ♦

## Your Gifts

Christina's comedy is relatable, and isn't it good to laugh? As she says, "being a human being is freaking ridiculous." Christina uses her gift to bring laughter and advocacy to women with a diagnosis.

What are your gifts? What skills, knowledge, and motivation can you use in your activism for mental health?

The second step on the Activism Path is to inventory your gifts to match them with activism opportunities. Exploring the gifts you bring to mental health activism allows you to increase the odds of success and maintain motivation.

Explore what you bring to the activism table.

### Your Skills

People often don't give themselves credit for their gifts and sometimes are not even aware of what they bring to the table. But we all have what author Mark Henson calls *ordinary superpowers.*[16] Mark recommends these questions to identify your superpowers.

*What do people say you do well?*

*What are you the go-to person for?*

Another good source to understand your gifts is to speak with someone you trust. Ask them what you do well. You might be surprised!

## Your Knowledge

Let's turn to what you know. Remind yourself of the knowledge you've gained just living your life.

Explore how and why you acquired this knowledge and whether you can translate it to activism.

### Mental Health Knowledge

You might be working in the mental health care field. You might have a diagnosis or simply acquired your knowledge as a family member or caregiver of someone with the lived experience. If you have a lot of knowledge or experience in an area, ask yourself how it can be used for the change you want to make in the world.

Let's assume you are new to mental health activism. In that case, this inventory will help you identify what knowledge you have and what you might need to obtain. Notice the types of publications, blogs, and podcasts you enjoy. What media do you watch? Which groups do you participate in? You might know more about mental health than you give yourself credit for.

### Check Your Cultural Competence

Activists need cultural competence to make an impact. Examine how you connect with those of diverse cultural backgrounds.

For example, understand your cultural biases and assumptions. What is your comfort level in dealing with others unlike you?

Broaden your understanding of other cultures to make your message more effective. Start with considering your background and culture and its impact on your attitudes and behavior.

Try to understand others' experiences when working together and avoid imposing your experiences on others.

Recognize where you hold privilege and how it affects your work. Pinpoint your areas of growth. With privilege comes advantages. For example, being White, male, Christian, heterosexual, upper-class, and English-speaking are advantages in the United States.

Your knowledge is vital to your success as an activist. So, take time to understand your gifts, cultural competence, and privilege.

## Clarify Your Motivation

"But what's in it for me?"

Is that a selfish question? No.

There's a lot of research on what motivates volunteers and activists, and the result is clear. You should ask yourself, "What's in it for me?" because if your activism work inspires you, it will get you through the tough times. And you'll stay with it longer. Effective long-term activists build motivation into their work.

Here are four areas of personal motivation.

### Translating Values into Positive Change

On the Activism Path, you clarify your values and passions for making change. The opportunity to translate those values and passions into activism work will motivate you.

New activist Heidi asked herself this question: What makes you angry? She found her activism passion in mental health care. She embraces the slogans "It's OK to not be OK" and "There's no health without mental health." Heidi is an outgoing extrovert, so she is comfortable openly sharing her opinions and concerns with people. She uses that gift to lobby her elected representatives on mental health legislation.

**Getting Satisfaction from the Activism Work Itself**

The pleasure from doing work is a powerful motivator. People motivated by the work itself are likely to work hard and push themselves to support a cause.

Jamie, a long-time mental health activist, found his pleasure volunteering as a suicide prevention counselor. But after a few years, he found the position was taking a toll on his own mental health. Jamie switched gears and became a freelance blogger specializing in suicide prevention education and mental health treatment. Jaime's writing is satisfying and has brought understanding and comfort to countless families who have read his blog posts online.

**Enjoying Working with Others**

Human beings have a built-in need to socialize. Activism with friends or family can be motivating, even if you are working on their cause rather than yours.

Amanda hasn't started working on her Activism Path, so she is unsure of the cause she is passionate about. But she knows she loves working with her best friend, Kathy, who advocates for reducing stigma toward those with mental illness. Kathy tells her own story of a mental health diagnosis and how the stigma made her afraid to seek help. Amanda is proud of Kathy for stepping out to tell her story, and she enjoys being with her. So, she chooses to support the mental health movement as her activism method. She acts as Kathy's assistant, scheduling, organizing, and traveling with her. Their time together brings them joy and their achievements bring them a mutual sense of purpose.

### Feeling Capable and Learning

Feeling capable motivates you. And as you achieve your goals for activism, your self-esteem will increase.

Jeffrey is a high school student who wants to improve mental health services for LGBTQ+ students. He doesn't have the same developed skill set as adult activists, but he wants to start working on the issue. By joining a group of LGBTQ+ activists, Jeffrey learns new skills. That way, he will better understand where his Activism Path will take him in the future.

## Want to Learn More?

We hope these activist stories have shown you the power of using your passion in a specific way to help others.

Take sufficient time for this step on the Activism Path. You will be more motivated and effective in your activism—and you might find your life is enhanced and fruitful in myriad ways.

At the end of each chapter, you will find additional resources for those who want the chance to get more detail about a topic.

If you are ready to move on, go to What's Next?

## Additional Resources

If you'd like help to inventory your skills, knowledge, and motivation, here are resources. These can help you in your work life, too.

1. To inventory your activism skills and knowledge, complete Randy Schutt's *Activist Skills and Experiences* questionnaire. The questionnaire is in *The What's On Your Sign? Workbook*, or at The Vernal Project.[17]
2. To better understand your privilege, try the *BuzzFeed* quiz "How Privileged Are You?"[18] We highly recommend it.
3. On the website *It's Pronounced Metrosexual*, you can find lists of situations that indicate you have privilege. For example, here is a list for those in the middle or upper-class.[19] One example: The "dream" of a house, a healthy family, and a solid career isn't a dream at all but simply a plan. We found this website enlightening.
4. Terri Lyon's books *What's On Your Sign?* and *The What's On Your Sign? Workbook* offer a structured approach to finding the perfect activism opportunity for you. One that makes a difference for those you love, doing something you love. Get exercises, worksheets, checklists, and reflective questions to help you identify your passion.

5. Visit Terri Lyon's website Life At The Intersection and start with the blog post "What You Can Do and What You Know Will Change The World."[20]

## What's Next?

Christina Wolfgram's story demonstrates a perfect match of her gift of humor with creative activism, which keeps her motivated while making people laugh.

But wait until you read Chapter 3. You'll see many activities that you never imagined could be used for activism. And hopefully, you will find the right one for you.

For example, how do quilting and activism go together? Read Karyl's story.

# CHAPTER 3

## MENTAL HEALTH ACTIVISM TECHNIQUES

**Start where you are. Use what you have. Do what you can.**

—ARTHUR ASHE

When you imagine activism, you might think of people protesting in the streets or speaking out from the steps of a governor's office. But that type of activism might not be your cup of tea.

The good news is there are many ways activists can make change. Using the Activism Path, you will find a match between your gifts and powerful motivation, like Karyl found after her daughter's death by suicide.

### Activist in Action: Karyl Chastain Beal

*Karyl Chastain Beal is not a well-known author, performer, speaker, social media influencer, or podcaster. She is a woman living in Spring Hill, Tennessee, who experienced her own pain and saw the pain of others and decided to turn a craft she loved into a key to open a locked door to a dark room and shine a desperately needed light.*

*Karyl talked with us about her own pain and grief and her choice to bring light and love to the reality of mental illness and suicide.*

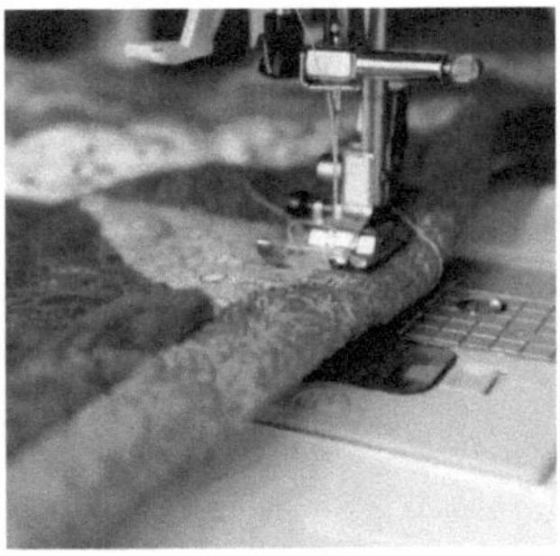

My daughter Arlyn died by suicide on August 7, 1996. She was diagnosed with bipolar disorder by a psychiatrist only after she died; based on her writings, we learned of her mental health struggles and of an apparent drug problem we knew nothing of.

Not only was I Arlyn's mother, but I was also a teacher. My ignorance on the issue of mental illness and the related drug abuse problem didn't cause her suicide, but my awareness and recognition of her issues before her death could possibly have changed the trajectory of her life.

Each year for the past fifteen years, I've coordinated the creation of a memorial quilt in honor of people who have died by suicide in Tennessee. The quilts accomplish a double mission.

First, people who are grieving the death of someone they love who died by suicide may be comforted to know that their loved ones will be remembered on a memorial quilt; since they know that the quilt will be displayed at suicide awareness and educational events, it may comfort them to know that their loved one's photo may help overcome the stigma associated with suicide and open a dialogue.

Second, the quilt helps educate the public about the fact that suicide happens to real people, people who were loved and valued—it's not cold hard data, they're not just statistics.

Generally, when people see a memorial quilt with a photo of their loved ones on it, they seem to be profoundly grateful.

It's hard to actually measure the impact long-term, but the immediate impact is obvious. When people see the quilt, they sometimes come to see it alone; other times, they bring a group of family members or friends with them because it's so important to them.

It's fairly common for people viewing the quilt to cry. Some of them sob. They don't take their eyes off of it. Many of them hug each other—or me. They take photos of the quilt and of themselves standing by the quilt. It's a memory they want to take with them. Seeing the memorial quilt is an experience they won't forget.

Mental health has always been in the closet, but it seems that if we crack the door open, some of the issues hidden in that small dark room will find their way out. Then, eventually, the world will be a healthier, happier, more peaceful place to live.

That's where I find the motivation to create the memorial quilts. I want to help others who walk the same road I've walked, but even more, I want to open the minds of other people to the fact that suicide prevention is essential and all lives are worth saving.

*View photos of the Love Never Dies quilts.*[21]

♦ ♦ ♦

## Traditional Approaches to Mental Health Activism

Karyl's story is about using a creative activism method, quilting. That is quite different from the traditional approaches to mental health activism: lobbying, advocacy, and fundraising. Although these approaches aren't quite as stimulating as others presented in this book, they are vital to the mental health community. So, if your gifts match these techniques, consider focusing on one.

### Advocacy (Educating Others)

Advocacy is essential to mental health awareness. Advocacy includes educating people about issues such as stigma. Advocacy is also used to welcome and prepare volunteers for activism work.

#### Educating Others

Examples:

The social media community includes many people with a diagnosis who share their stories to reduce the stigma of mental illness. If you enjoy interacting on social media, consider this technique.

- ✓ Stand up for others by sharing your story privately with a friend, neighbor, or loved one. You also don't have to share your story if you're not yet ready. Both NAMI and MHA suggest that you:
    - ⇒ Support someone who needs help
    - ⇒ Volunteer for a local mental health organization

⇒ Attend an awareness walk or other event benefiting the mental health movement

⇒ Encourage your local politicians to prioritize mental health

⇒ Correct those who use stigmatizing language

✓ Nonprofits welcome volunteers but getting them up to speed takes time and effort. If you are an excellent teacher, support mental health awareness by helping prepare volunteers for their work.

✓ Organizations put on awareness days to focus attention on mental health. Volunteer at community events related to mental health, like health fairs, health resource events, and parenting fairs.

**Patient and Family Support Programs**

Mental health organizations provide support programs for those with a diagnosis and their caregivers. NAMI, Mental Health America (MHA), and the American Foundation for Suicide Prevention (AFSP) are just three of the national organizations that offer support groups for those with the lived experience and their families and caregivers.

Examples:

✓ Work with your local NAMI affiliate, join an affiliate board/steering committee or become an instructor for NAMI programs like Family-to-Family[22].

- ✓ NAMI Smarts for Advocacy[23] is a hands-on advocacy training program. People living with mental illness and their friends and families transform their passion and lived experience into skillful grassroots advocacy.
- ✓ MHA seeks motivated volunteers to support their events, such as mental health screenings, and take part in their legislative advocacy efforts.
- ✓ Mental Health First Aid[24] is an eight-hour course that teaches you how to help someone experiencing a mental health or substance use challenge. The training enables you to identify, understand, and respond to signs of addictions and mental illnesses.
- ✓ Become a volunteer for the National Suicide Prevention Lifeline.[25]

**Community Support Programs**

Be a resource to those in the community with mental illness.

Examples:

- ✓ Work to bring Crisis Intervention Team training to your community. This team supports law enforcement to help those experiencing a mental health crisis.
- ✓ The QPR Institute uses a simple three-step process of Question-Persuade-Refer[26] to save lives and reduce suicidal behaviors. QPR training is available in hundreds of cities across the US and can be taken online.

- ✓ The MakeItOK[27] campaign is designed to reduce stigma. The website offers extensive resources, such as posters, flyers, a PowerPoint presentation, brochures, tip cards, and more.
- ✓ Help prevent suicide in the elderly population by using social opportunities to combat isolation.

## Lobbying

Lobbying is talking to people in government who have influence over your issue. Your goal is to state your position on the subject and persuade the other person to use their power on your behalf.

Examples:

- ✓ Meet with your state representative to ask for better access to mental health care in your community.
- ✓ Call your senator to ask for changes to Medicare options.

## Fundraising

Fundraising is an essential task in activism. Your community connections can pay off in financial support for mental health organizations. Funding is desperately needed for improvements to mental health care and treatment. Consider becoming involved in these ways.

Examples:

- ✓ Participate in NAMIWalks, an annual 5K (3.1 miles) walk to promotes awareness about mental illness and raise funds for NAMI state chapters and local affiliates.

And we can say from experience, it is a fun and joyous experience.

- ✓ Have a Facebook fundraiser, a simple way to request donations to the nonprofit organization of your choice. Folks have fundraisers for birthdays, graduations, and for any life event. So why not raise money to support a mental health organization?
- ✓ Have your garden club sell bouquets and donate the proceeds to a mental health charity.
- ✓ Create a product that highlights mental health awareness and donate the proceeds to your cause. Brewers Dave and Emily Mobley donate the proceeds of a beer called "Your Story Is Not Complete"[28] to a suicide prevention organization in honor of Dave's brother Josh, who died by suicide.

## Rallies

With rallies and public events, organizers hope to increase awareness and change public opinion about mental illness.

Examples:

- ✓ Attend a rally day at your state capital to influence elected officials.
- ✓ Organize a public event in your town to bring awareness to the difficulties faced by people living with mental illness, as NAMI Chattanooga (Tennessee) did. NAMI Narratives: Finding Courage in Mental Illness, is an

outdoor event in which courageous community members impacted by mental illness share their stories with the public to destigmatize mental illness and promote open and honest conversation.

### Summary

Lobbying, advocacy, and fundraising are necessary types of mental health activism. If you enjoy these activities, please use your skills to support those with mental illness and their caregivers. But if these methods don't motivate you, read on, because there are other ways you can make a difference.

## Creative Approaches to Mental Health Activism

Now, for those of you who don't want to lobby elected officials, teach, or fundraise, you can still make a difference doing something you love.

### The Arts

Putting the arts and activism together sounds strange, doesn't it? But many professional and amateur artists use their skills for social justice, like Karyl and Christinea. Why not apply your talents to mental health awareness?

#### Drawing and Illustration

Do you have the ability to draw, illustrate, sculpt or paint? Use your skills to make a difference.

Examples:

- ✓ Create a mental health T-shirt design.
- ✓ Organize a drawing contest for mental health awareness and fundraising.
- ✓ Create art to display in your community. Artist Kimmy Henderson installs sculpted butterflies in her communities to highlight bipolar awareness.[29]
- ✓ Offer art therapy classes to those with a diagnosis.
- ✓ Do portraits of famous mental health advocates. (Get inspired by Joan Baez, who created an exhibition of well-known activists.[30])

**Crafting**

Are you a crafter? If you love to knit, crochet, or embroider, use your skills for mental health awareness.

Examples:

- ✓ Embroider a message about mental health on a handkerchief and send it to your elected representative. (Hat tip to the Craftivist Collective31 for this idea.)
- ✓ Sew mental health-related shirts for stuffed teddy bears.
- ✓ Knitters can handcraft mental health messages and display them in a well-visited spot in their community.

**Theater**

The theater, like film, impacts social change by using a compelling story. It displays a live, three-dimensional message more powerful than movies because of the immediacy and intimate setting.

If you love theater, think about ways you can use your passion for mental health awareness.

Examples:

- ✓ An innovative theater group called Acting for The Future hosts "participative drama workshops, professional performances and post-show panel discussions with counselors and clinical psychologists to promote active healthy lifestyles, positive mental health, and suicide prevention."[32]
- ✓ Pair up with a clinical psychologist to provide a participative workshop, where attendees can practice ways to maintain their mental health.
- ✓ Ask theater companies to mount productions focused on mental illness.
- ✓ Write a play about stigma for your high school.

**Music**

Music is a beautiful way to reach people. It can be used to inspire, relax, or rouse people to action.

For example, rapper Logic used his talent in the song "1-800-273-8255 (National Suicide Prevention Lifeline)." According to

Vibrant Emotional Health, formerly the Mental Health Association of New York City (MHA-NYC), in a December 2017 article on its website:

*Thanks to the heightened public awareness of the Lifeline due to increased media and National Suicide Prevention Month, as well as a general increase in call volume compared to last year, the Lifeline experienced its highest-ever call volume during September 2017. After Logic's performance at the Video Music Awards [September 2017], the Lifeline saw a 50% increase in call volume in the hours after the show. Since the song's release, the Lifeline website has also gained an extra 100,000 visitors per month.*[33]

In a press release from Vibrant, Logic says,

*In [this song] we hear a person at the end of their rope. . . . We then hear words from the perspective of the Lifeline counselor who in turn gives them many reasons to keep fighting for their life. . . . Finally, we hear the caller express their new lease on life and outlook on a life that they thought was over but had actually been far from it all along.*[34]

Examples:

- ✓ Set poems about mental illness to music.
- ✓ Create a playlist for someone who is a caregiver.
- ✓ Write a song about mental illness and perform it at an open mic night.

**Writing**

Perhaps you have a way with words. There are many ways you can use this talent to help those with a diagnosis and their caregivers.

Pete Earley has a way with words, and it paid off for at least one person. One man with mental illness sought help at a mental health center, and, in his pocket, they found one of Pete's op-eds from *USA Today*. The man's mother wrote to Pete, saying the article helped encourage her son to seek treatment.

Examples:

- ✓ Ask people to contribute song lyrics, poetry, and essays to a collection.
- ✓ Start a blog about mental health issues and include activist profiles and interviews.
- ✓ Share your experiences with mental illness on social media and create a support community.
- ✓ Write an article about mental illness in your community for your newspaper.
- ✓ Write a memoir about your lived experiences with mental illness.

**Photography**

Photos can inspire and educate us. If you are a shutterbug, how can you contribute?

Examples:

- ✓ Create a book of photos of those with a diagnosis.
- ✓ Teach photography to those with a diagnosis.
- ✓ Start an Instagram account to share your experiences with mental illness.

- ✓ Contribute photos about mental illness to media outlets.

## Specialized Skills

### Leadership

A lack of skilled leaders hinders most activist organizations. Without enough leaders, they end up tabling work important to their movement. They need leaders who can communicate a vision, inspire performance toward a goal, recruit and develop volunteers, and make change happen.

Examples:

- ✓ Reconsider work in the for-profit sector and consider a nonprofit job in mental health.
- ✓ Offer to use your strategic planning skills to help a nonprofit improve its operations.
- ✓ Run volunteer motivation and engagement sessions.

### Legal Support

People with a legal background are much needed in mental health activism.

Examples:

- ✓ The MHA Advocacy Network[35] includes thousands of people who actively protect America's mental health through legislative advocacy.
- ✓ Volunteer in your community's Legal Aid to help people with diagnoses.

### News Media Outreach

Activist organizations use news media outreach to give information about the cause to a broad audience. One way to make an impact is to develop relationships with reporters who write about your cause. Pitch them a story about how your activism relates to mental health, and you might get a feature article in your local newspaper.

Examples:

- ✓ Connect personally with someone at your local newspaper. Send well-written articles about mental health issues regularly.
- ✓ Ask the editor to run a regular mental health-related column.

## Movement Support

In the same way leaders can help others use their strengths, those in movement support can take care of others' tasks. Supporting others in the movement can multiply the impact of the activism community.

### Caregiving

This work supports most activism efforts. Provide support so volunteers, employees, and caregivers don't have to worry about other areas of their lives while helping the cause.

Examples:

- ✓ Create a referral program of people who would offer free or discounted help with personal needs. This might include home repairs, transportation, caregiver days out, and caregiver meetups where food is prepared and served free of charge.

- ✓ Offer yoga or meditation classes to those with a diagnosis or to caregivers.
- ✓ Provide food and drink for caregiver support classes.

**Administrative Work**

This work supports most activism efforts. Every movement has tasks that just have to be done, such as setting up computers, answering correspondence, and handling money.

Examples:

- ✓ Make copies and help set up for a mental health forum.
- ✓ Volunteer for tasks at your state mental health convention.
- ✓ Manage the AV equipment for your local mental health organization's events.

## It's not Slacktivism: Activism for People with Limited Time

You want to make a difference, but you also have a job, family, and limited time. If this is true, the following section highlighting quick activism is for you.

**Social Media: Podcasts/ Social Media Campaigns**

The internet has changed activism. Whether that change is directly making a difference in a cause is still unknown. But there is no denying the power of social media to connect with like-minded others and organize and implement social change activities.

**Radio, Video, and Podcasts**

Examples:

- ✓ Offer to do local radio interviews about your experiences.
- ✓ Create a YouTube channel to speak on mental health issues. Interview those with a diagnosis as well as caregivers, physicians, advocates, and politicians.
- ✓ Do a podcast or be interviewed on the podcasts of others.
- ✓ Man Therapy: Manly Mental Health Tips[36] uses a unique blend of humor and evidence to help men learn how to better talk about their mental health issues—and get the help they need. Humor is the key. Check out the episode about how men do yoga as proof.

**Social Media**

Examples:

- ✓ Create a local Facebook page to promote NAMI activities, training, classes, and news.
- ✓ #CureStigma and the StigmaFree Pledge[37] are NAMI's social media campaigns to stop stigma.

- ✓ Use digital communication to help provide crucial support and services to those suffering from mental health issues. Big White Wall[38] is an example. They support members in self-managing their care.

## Corporate Protests

Corporate protests have increased as activists use their buying power to advocate for change within companies. This has led businesses to see employees, shareholders, and activist groups as stakeholders and recognize their viewpoints in company decisions.

### Employee Activism

Example:

- ✓ Speak up at work if your company allows the use of mental illness-related words such as *crazy* or *insane* to refer to anything negative, different, or difficult. Instead, gently suggest they substitute a similar word, such as *wild* or *ridiculous,* that does not contribute to stigma toward those with the lived experience.

### Shareholder Activism

Shareholder activism is a form of corporate boycott by those who own shares in the company. A bloc of shareholders voting together can influence the company to change policies and practices.

Examples:

- ✓ Shareholders can protest companies that do not provide a living wage. Having sufficient resources to live on contributes to mental health.
- ✓ Shareholders can ask for better benefits and unpenalized time off for those who need treatment.
- ✓ Shareholders can ask for better benefits and unpenalized time off for those who care for a family member with a diagnosis.

**Consumer Activism: Boycotts and Buycotts**

Have you boycotted any products because you disagree with the company's stance on an issue? *Buycotts* are the opposite—support an organization by purchasing their products. Both can make a difference.

Examples:

- ✓ In 1999, NAMI protested the Nestlé food company for the stigmatized names of their Taffy Bars: *Psycho Sam*, *Looney Jerry*, and *Weird Wally*.
- ✓ Wear your support for mental health awareness. A wide variety of clothing and accessories promote awareness. Green ribbon lapel pins are worn to represent support for mental health. Be prepared to address the issue and answer questions.
- ✓ Boycott companies that discriminate against those with a diagnosis or their caregivers.

- ✓ Activist Liz Beecroft and Nike created the Air Max 270 React *In My Feels* shoe to support mental health awareness.[39]

**Petitions**

Petitions are floating around on many topics; signing them is an easy and effective way to participate in this type of activism.

Examples:

- ✓ Change.org has many petitions about mental health. The site also contains tools to create your own petitions.
- ✓ Create a petition to support the mental health of local teachers.
- ✓ Does your local high school have a gay–straight alliance (GSA)? If not, create a petition to start one.

## Summary

We hope this section on creative activism techniques has sparked ideas for how you can use your gifts for mental health awareness. Get creative!

## The Right Activism Method for You

As you learned here, there are so many activism methods, so many choices.

Karyl uses her quilting skills to help those in grief commemorate their loved ones who died by suicide. And in doing so, she educates others.

When you consider your gifts and motivation, how do they match up with either the traditional activism methods or the creative techniques?

What activism methods made you feel energized? Did something call to you?

We hope these activist stories have shown you the power of using your passion in a specific way to help those with mental illness.

## Want to Learn More?

Take sufficient time for this step on the Activism Path. You will be more motivated and effective in your activism—and you might find your life is enhanced and fruitful in myriad ways.

At the end of each chapter, you will find additional resources for those who want the chance to get more detail about a topic.

If you are ready to move on, go to What's Next?

### Additional Resources

If you'd like to learn more about activism methods, here are resources.

1. Terri Lyon's books *What's On Your Sign?* and *The What's On Your Sign? Workbook* offer a structured approach to finding the perfect activism opportunity for you. One that makes a difference for those you love, doing something you love. Get exercises, worksheets, checklists, and reflective questions to help you the best activism method for you.

2. Visit Terri's website Life At The Intersection and start with the blog post "How to Find The Best Activism Method."[40]

## What's Next?

The next chapter is about making the most impact possible for mental health.

You'll meet Miana Bryant, an activist calling out the elephant in the room: stigma. By doing so, she makes an impact on behalf of college students with a mental health diagnosis.

# CHAPTER 4

## ACTIVISM THAT MAKES AN IMPACT

**In a gentle way, you can shake the world.**

—MAHATMA GANDHI

Of course, you want to make the biggest splash possible with your mental health activism. With so many ways to make a difference in the world, make sure you check whether your activism really works and is the right personal fit for you. Will your work change lives? Evaluating your effectiveness is not an easy step, but it is worth the effort.

Activist in Action Miana Bryant wants to eliminate the stigma of mental illness. Her organization, The Mental Elephant, is named based on the expression *the elephant in the room*, which means an important topic, question, or controversial issue that is obvious or that everyone knows about, but no one mentions or wants to discuss. But by talking about it, Miana makes life a little easier for college students with a mental health diagnosis.

The Mental Elephant [41] provides support groups, engagement events, and study sessions for students with a diagnosis. This safe place allows participants who worry about stigma to talk about their diagnosis.

NAMI Chief Medical Officer Dr. Ken Duckworth, who wrote the Afterword for this book, said on *CBS This Morning* in October 2019,

*Miana's generation is changing this game. We are at a tipping point in our society. . . . Young women [like Miana] are tipping the scales away from stigma and toward openness and vulnerability.*[42]

## Activist in Action: Miana Bryant

*Miana Bryant is, by any measure, a remarkable young woman. She holds a bachelor of arts in psychology and criminal justice from East Carolina University (ECU). Miana's life and career plans took an unexpected turn when, in her early teens, she was diagnosed with depression and anxiety. Adolescence is hard enough, but her struggle was life altering. Bryant took her mental health challenges and created something good—The Mental Elephant, which you can find on Instagram, YouTube, and Facebook.*

*She is the sole founder and currently the only editor of all online outlets. Aside from online work, she is also the president of The Mental Elephant Organization. We asked Miana to tell us about her activism.*

It is important for me to advocate on behalf of mental health because mental health education and support are not focused enough in [underrepresented] populations that so desperately need it. Mental health is the foundation of production for all humans and needs to be handled the same as physical health.

Of my many objectives, the two most important to me are my desire to implement mental health treatment resources in low-income areas, and to work to bring mental health training to law enforcement agencies.

There is so much to do. I don't focus on how many people I've helped, more so on who's next. I like to think that I've impacted people I've met and those who know of me through other channels.

Here is what I would love everyone to know—it's okay to struggle and not know what's going on. I'm 24 years old, living with my parents again, constantly in a state of confusion. And it's okay. I tell myself as I tell others, focus on getting to the next moment and doing what you can with what you have. Don't harp on things out of our control. The world is currently a stressful place with people losing hope daily. It's important to focus on how to help yourself within the moment.

♦ ♦ ♦

Miana's story reminds us that life can come at you fast. Still, even challenges can present opportunities to be of service to others. Miana turned her passion into concrete activism that has helped hundreds of college students.

*I know that there are going to be days where you think your world is collapsing, there's going to be moments where you're not even sure how you are going to get through the next sixty seconds. The only thing you, on this Earth, 100% have to do is breathe.*

## Your Activism Opportunities

You are at step 4 on the Activism Path! Here you will use your work on the previous steps to bring it all together and identify your mental health activism opportunities—opportunities that make an impact and are the right personal fit for you.

For some people, like Miana, the match between their gifts and activism opportunities is easy to see. But most people need a process to find their match. Brainstorming ideas about how to best use your gifts can lead to ideas you might never have unearthed without creative thinking.

You will choose the type of activism experiences that best suit you. Then you will narrow down your options. The work you've done so far will guide you to the right activism opportunities.

### Steps to Finding Activism Opportunities

In step 1, you considered your passions. Step 2 required you to inventory your gifts. In step 3, you found activism methods that light your fire.

Now, brainstorm activism options and whittle them down to your top three. Ask yourself, which one of these will have the most impact?

## Brainstorm Your Options

Fortunately, there are several methods you can use to brainstorm your activism opportunities.

### Intersections

Here is our favorite method to find your activism options. Intersections. No, not the traffic kind, but the Venn diagrammy kind.

Identify any combination of gifts, methods, and motivators. Use these to create overlapping circles with a place in the center that is common to all three. That is where you will look for activism opportunities. The intersection of three circles leads to creative options.

Intersections are helpful when you have multiple gifts or are interested in several different methods.

If you have multiple interests, look for the intersection of those interests to find where you can make a unique contribution.

### Examples of Using Intersections

In our first example, a woman likes to teach and draw, and she wants to help victims of racism. What work is possible for her cause? Perhaps she can teach a course on helping victims of racism tell their stories through art.

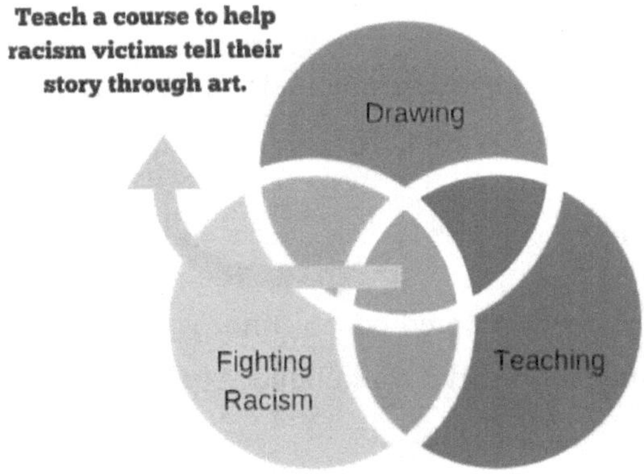


Someone else might use Planning (skill), Art (skill), and Advocacy (method) in her intersection. From this, she came up with the idea to create an artistic calendar focused on mental health awareness. It will include important dates, reminders from events in history, training opportunities, and resources.

A third person used different categories in his intersection: Social Media (method), Fundraising (method), and Enjoying Working with Others (motivator.) This helped him decide to create an online fundraiser where you tag someone and ask them to donate for a person in their lives who has a diagnosis.

You will find a blank intersection worksheet on the Mental Health Activism Companion Website. Try different combinations and let your creativity guide you.

If this isn't a method that works for you, try starting with your skills.

### Your Skills and Activism Method Choice

Another way to evaluate your activism opportunities is to reflect on your best skill and how to apply it to mental health activism, as shown below.

- ✓ If you are skilled in influencing others, advocate for examining different mental health outcomes by race.
- ✓ If you can create a strategic vision, plan a campaign for a mental health-friendly candidate to run for office.
- ✓ If you like to make movies, create a documentary about a caregiver's experience with stress.
- ✓ If you enjoy the theater, write a play about how mental illness impacts families.
- ✓ If you understand journalism and news outreach, research which journalists regularly write about mental health and connect with them.
- ✓ If you don't mind a good protest, sit-in at your elected representative's office to support having trained professionals respond to mental health calls instead of law enforcement

## Narrow Your Options with a Focus on Impact

Now that you have listed activism opportunities, evaluate them to determine which will have the most impact.

The criteria we use are based on the *effective altruism movement*, a process to determine which charities get the biggest bang for their buck.

For your activism opportunities, consider:

1. Will the activism dramatically improve a large number of lives?
2. How much change can you make?
3. How much is the method overlooked?
4. Will my gifts and passions lead to making a difference?

## 1. Will the Activism Dramatically Improve a Large Number of Lives?

This is an excellent place to start your evaluation since making a difference for the greatest number of people is usually the best option.

## 2. How Much Change Can You Make?

This evaluation takes a bit more thought. Some types of activism can make a great deal of change, while other types might not. For example, Miana Bryant's activism for college students with a diagnosis made a considerable difference.

Whereas efforts to get law enforcement with crisis intervention team (CIT) training to respond to mental health crisis calls might be hampered by a lack of CIT trained officers in your area.

### 3. How Much Is the Method Overlooked?

Some activism opportunities receive a great deal of attention, while others don't. Where might your efforts make more of a difference? For Miana, focusing on supporting and educating college students was a no-brainer because there were no resources, tools, and materials available at her school.

### 4. Will My Gifts and Passions Lead to Making a Difference?

Finally, and perhaps most importantly, will your passion and gifts lead to real change? A great personal fit of your skills and motivation with a cause you love means better engagement and results.

## Want to Learn More?

Take sufficient time for this step on the Activism Path. You will be more motivated and effective in your activism—and you might find your life is enhanced and fruitful in myriad ways.

Below are additional resources for those who want the chance to get more detail about a topic.

If you are ready to move on, go to What's Next?

### Additional Resources

If you'd like help brainstorming activism opportunities and evaluating their impact, here are resources.

1. *What's On Your Sign?* and *The What's On Your Sign? Workbook* offer a structured approach to finding the perfect activism opportunity for you. Get exercises, worksheets, checklists, and reflective questions to help you complete the process.
2. Visit Terri's website Life At The Intersection and start with the blog post "How To Make An Impact with Your Activism."[43]
3. Read *Doing Good Better*[44] by William MacAskill to learn how to make a difference with your charitable donations.

## What's Next?

You are at step 5, the final step of the Activism Path. This is where you set yourself up for success. Learn how activist Gabe Howard uses tenacity and professionalism to help those—like himself—with mental illness.

# CHAPTER 5

## YOUR ACTION PLAN TO STAY MOTIVATED

**Change will not come if we wait for some other person or some other time. We are the ones we've been waiting for. We are the change that we seek.**

—BARACK OBAMA, FORMER PRESIDENT

In this chapter, you will set yourself up for success in your activism. First, set goals to stay focused and motivated for your work. Then, learn to recognize how your body responds to stress so you can manage your reactions. Finally, you'll celebrate your accomplishments. Activist Gabe Howard says tenacity is vital for those in activism—and how sometimes you have to take a deep breath before you go on.

### Activist in Action: Gabe Howard

*Gabe Howard*[45] *is a bit of a Renaissance man in the world of mental health activism. He is an award-winning speaker, author, and podcaster who lives with bipolar disorder. He hosts the weekly podcast* Inside Mental Health. *His popular book on the challenges of living with bipolar disorder is boldly titled* Mental Illness is an Asshole and Other Observations. *And that, friends, tells you a lot about Gabe Howard.*

*We asked Gabe why he so publicly talks about his mental illness.*

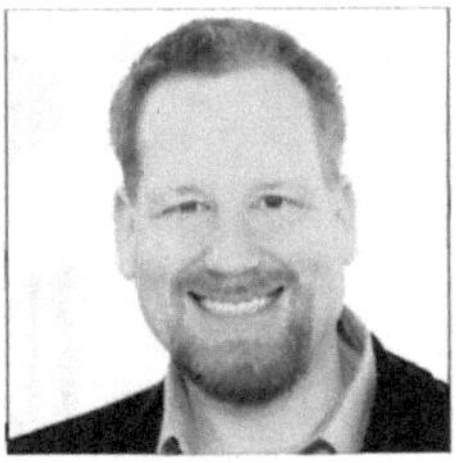

Because my experience was terrible and it didn't need to be. I could have gotten help much sooner. My family didn't have to suffer like they did. I just realized that someone needs to fix this and while I don't believe I can do it all by myself, I did (and do) believe that I have a role to play. I just don't want the next person to go through what I went through.

What I'd like to see happen is for everyone with mental illness to be treated the same. It's not lost on me that being a White middle-class guy in a big city with health insurance, money, and strong family support meant that I got better and faster care. That's not fair. I want everyone to understand the warning signs. I want everyone to have access to care.

I also realized that people only see mental illness as a crisis—crisis is very public. News broadcasts and social media play a role in this. I want to ensure that society sees people with a mental health diagnosis living well. If all people ever see is crisis and suffering then no one will believe that they can get well. That's a terrible thing, in my opinion. We must have hope.

When I'm asked about how effective I think my work is, I have to admit that, sadly, I don't have access to the tools that would give me excellent data. For me, I judge it by the number of people who listen to my podcasts, my social media traffic, and my email box. I also judge my success or failure by what people say to me after a speech, presentation, or when I'm at a conference or meeting. I truly try to keep the lines of communication open and let people tell me what's on their mind—the good, the bad, and the ugly.

Regarding my book, I wrote it to let readers know that I worked really hard to reach recovery with bipolar disorder, but that I did not do it alone. I had the help of doctors, peers, family, and, frankly, I had luck. I was lucky to have access to health care and I was lucky someone noticed I was struggling and took me to the emergency room. That person saved my life. No one can beat mental illness alone. I really believe that.

Activism work is indescribably rewarding. But buckle up! It's a slow process that is filled with more setbacks than anything. Tenacity matters—but so does professionalism. If you choose to be a mental health activist that means that when someone says something offensive, awful, or stigmatizing your job is to help them understand why stigma is not cool. I understand the urge to scold people, but that's not advocacy. That's revenge. Take a deep breath and explain your feelings and the feelings of all of us. You will create a safe space to answer questions and have a much-needed conversation. That's the only way forward.

Believe me, if yelling at people would solve this problem, it would already be solved. Because I have a big, loud mouth!

◆ ◆ ◆

## Your Action Plan

Gabe's story reminds us it is essential to have goals, persevere, and stay calm. Even if you have a big personality! He also reminds us how rewarding the work can be.

By following the Activism Path, you have made inroads into finding the best activism opportunity to support mental health. Congratulations!

In this chapter, you will create an action plan to help you get started on the right foot.

If you are not quite to the point where you know your activism opportunity, that's fine too. Some people need more time than others to decide the best match for them. Thoughtful reflection will increase your odds of being effective and staying motivated. Take your time.

When you are ready, come back here to create your action plan.

## Create Your Action Plan

Your action plan will include:

- ✓ goal setting,
- ✓ stress awareness,
- ✓ checking in and refocusing, if necessary, and
- ✓ celebrating your accomplishments.

## Activism Goals

Setting goals for your activism will make you more effective. Lots of research supports this.

Goals and goal setting have become trendy terms in recent years. But don't let the media overload of these terms turn you off. Goal setting is a vital component of any successful long-term endeavor. Without clear goals, you are more likely to stray from your intended activism target. Goals that are too general or too specific can hinder your success also. Timelines that are too rushed or too far in the future invite failure. The key is to find the right balance. The ultimate goal is a clear, doable action plan.

An internet search for goal-setting methods will help you find the technique that works best for you. But here is an article that offers excellent advice and several interactive, printable templates to aid you in this part of finding success and motivation for your mental health activism: The Easy Guide to the Goal-setting Process.[46]

Take time to set specific goals for yourself. Skipping this process might save time now, but will cost you time and achievement in the future.

## Self-Care Stress Awareness

Activism can bring opportunities for stress. You might be in conflict with people who believe differently. Perhaps you stress about not accomplishing enough. In some activism, you might feel unsafe. You might have less time with your family.

Learn what stress symptoms appear in your body to head off stress while it is still manageable.

The Mental Health Activism Companion Website includes a checklist from Baylor University to rate your overall stress level.

Coping strategies help you head off stress before it becomes overwhelming. Consider using one or more of these coping strategies when you experience stress.

- ✓ Use the people in your life as a support network.
- ✓ Control your reactions to events by training your mind to interpret them in a more rational, positive way.
- ✓ Incorporate gratefulness into your work

## Refocusing

If the need to choose a different focus altogether arises, go back to the Activism Path work you've done and see what other direction your passion takes you. Work the process so you are still using your skills and knowledge, are motivated, and make the change you want in the world.

## Celebration

Our experience with activists is that they are caring people who tend to think about others more than themselves. This passion for service is a beautiful thing.

But remember that you want to make a difference for a long time. To do that, you must understand what motivates you and build that into your work. Remember, you did this in step 2 when you identified your personal motivation and made that a part of your activism.

When you accomplish something, like one of your goals, reward yourself.

We've learned that activists would rather use their money for their cause instead of themselves. But, think about rewarding yourself as an investment in your cause—something that motivates you by reminding you of what you've accomplished.

- ✓ Recognize yourself for the work you have done to make the change you want in the world. Even a small reward will be affirming.
- ✓ Try something that makes you feel pampered and reduces your stress, like a massage.
- ✓ A lovely reward that links you to the essential people in your life is a meal with a friend.
- ✓ Remind yourself how wonderful you are to make a difference for people with a diagnosis and their caregivers.

## Want to Learn More?

Take sufficient time for this step on the Activism Path. You will be more motivated and effective in your activism—and you might find your life is enhanced and fruitful in myriad ways.

Below are additional resources for those who want the chance to get more detail about a topic.

If you are ready to move on, go to What's Next?

### Additional Resources

If you'd like help with your action plan, here are resources.

1. Read The Lifelong Activist: How to change the world without losing your way by Hillary Rettig.[47]
2. Use a guide for writing SMART goals provided by the University of California.[48]
3. Read 11 Change-Makers Share How They Deal with Activism Fatigue.[49]
4. Learn how to incorporate gratefulness into your life.[50]
5. Try Savor Your Life: A Tool for Boosting Happiness.[51]
6. Complete a Stress Test from PsychCentral.[52]
7. Terri Lyon's books *What's On Your Sign?* and *The What's On Your Sign? Workbook* offer a structured approach to finding the perfect activism opportunity for you. One that makes a difference for those you love, doing something you love. Get exercises, worksheets, checklists, and reflective questions to help you the best activism method for you.
8. Visit Terri's website Life At The Intersection and start with the blog post "How To Stay Motivated in Your Activism."[53]

## What's Next?

You're ready!

# CONCLUSION

## YOU CAN BE A MENTAL HEALTH ACTIVIST

**The problem with mental illness is people don't look at it as a physical illness. When you think about it, the brain is actually the most complex organ in your body. We need to treat it like a physical illness and take it seriously.**

—DEMI LOVATO[54]

Yes, you can be a mental health activist. With this book, we have fulfilled our desire to prepare you to make a difference for those with mental health disorders, those who love them, and our communities in general.

## What You Learned from the Activism Path

Here is a reminder of all you learned about getting started in activism:

1. Focus your passion for mental health.
2. Match your skills with the type of activism work that best suits you.
3. Find an activism opportunity that works for your life.

4. Determine if your mental health activism truly makes an impact.
5. Stay motivated in your activism for the long term.

If you have worked through these five steps, you are better prepared than most people who start in activism.

So—what are you waiting for?

## Tips from the Activists in Action

We asked our wonderful Activists in Action what advice they have for new mental health activists.

### Your Passion

In step 1 of the Activism Path, you are focused on your passion. Karyl Chastain Beal recommends you help others find their unique way to support mental health awareness.

Pete Earley wants you to tap your passion when the going gets tough:

*Speaking out is not easy. Dealing with someone with a serious mental illness is not easy. But know that what you are doing is going to help save lives. You will be giving a voice to those who often go unheard or unseen.*

### Your Gifts

Step 2 of the Activism Path had you inventory your gifts to use in your activism.

Christinea Beane's activism started with a care package to a total stranger and built into a jewelry business that stimulates conversation and generates mental illness awareness. She found that using her artistic talent was the perfect match for her. She recommends that you make sure you have the qualifications or skills needed for your activism.

Our activists' words and results clearly show that they are all strongly motivated by one thing. They translate their values into positive change.

## Your Activism Opportunity

In step 3, you find activism opportunities that motivate you and work in your life.

Our activists followed their passion and used their skills to find the right activism opportunity. They tapped their creative sides: Christinea and Karyl with crafting, Christina and Gabe with podcasting, and Pete with writing.

Karyl reminds us that we want to go out and save the world after a tragedy. Although we may be motivated, we may not be ready yet:

*As the flight attendants tell us, put your own face mask on first. You can't help others until you're safe.*

## Your Impact

As a prominent mental health activist, Pete has seen what works and recommends these programs for their impact:

- ✓ Crisis Intervention Team (CIT) Training

- ✓ Pre- and post-jail diversion
- ✓ Mental health dockets
- ✓ Mobile crisis response teams
- ✓ Drop off centers rather than emergency rooms and jails
- ✓ Greater use of peers
- ✓ More sensible laws that allow intervention before imminent danger
- ✓ Housing solutions
- ✓ Crisis care beds
- ✓ Longer-term beds for those who need more than a few days to be properly diagnosed and offered treatment
- ✓ Housing First
- ✓ Assertive Community Treatment (ACT) teams that offers individually tailored services can effectively help most individuals with mental illnesses recovery

Pete wants to see the cost of jailing a mentally ill person used for these impactful programs:[55]

*For half that, we could provide housing and an ACT team and help someone recover rather than condemning them to the streets, jails, back on streets, jail treadmill. Just as putting a human face on mental illnesses helps humanize the illness and fight stigma, having a treatment team that has a personal relationship with someone who is sick is essential to helping them recover. How do we achieve this?*

*By proving that wrap-around services save lives and, in most cases, save money.*

*To make the most impact on young people, Miana recommends staying up to date with the ways young people communicate, such as the latest apps.*

*The best ways to reach people are through methods and technology they already use and understand.*

It is no surprise that step 4, evaluating impact, is the most difficult one for our activists. They admit they don't have formal ways to measure their impact. But our activists are united about the best feedback on their impact. They know they are on the right path when someone they helped contacts them. As Pete says:

*The real measure of success is when someone with a mental illness or a loved one of someone with a mental illness tells me that they either heard my son or me give a speech or read something that I had written and it helped them.*

## Your Motivation

Step 5 showed you how to plan, set goals, and manage your stress. Karyl provided several tips for this step. She recommends a step-by-step plan with goals and timelines. In addition, she believes that anticipating roadblocks improves impact and reduces stress:

*Find a support system to help you. The support system can include friends, family members, professionals, others who share the same mission, and cheerleaders.*

## Pete's Seven Biggest Takeaways

Pete Earley has given this matter a great deal of thought. Here are Pete's words to inspire you to play a role in making a difference with mental health activism and stay the course:

First, mental illnesses are serious business. You can't take an aspirin and wake up in the morning healed. It took more than five years for my son to become stable. Parents and others need to realize that there are no quick fixes. Hang in there and realize there will be many highs and lows on your journey.

Second, accept a new normal. Saying you want your child to go back to the way he was is counterproductive. You need to understand that the person you love has a mental illness. Most people can and do recover. But the journey that you go through with them to recovery changes both of you. There is no going back to the past.

Third, learn to trust your own judgment. No one knows the person you love better than you, and while there are amazing, devoted, and really smart mental health professionals, they do not have to live with the person who is sick. You must be resilient. Trust your heart.

Fourth, educate yourself. Think of mental illness as a formidable enemy and realize you need to be knowledgeable to prevent it from destroying your loved one's life.

Join a national mental health group, such as NAMI or Mental Health America. Learn about CIT training and find out if law enforcement in your community has CIT officers who you can call.

Become knowledgeable about medications and alternatives. Obtain the tools that you need to help someone you love.

Fifth, realize that mental illnesses impact your entire family. Siblings often are jealous of all the attention that is being shown to someone with a disorder. They accuse their troubled brother or sister of acting out to get attention or of manipulating their parents. Encouraging them to learn about mental illness and including them in helping someone recover can ease those feelings.

Sixth, understand your own limitations. This is perhaps the most difficult lesson to learn. Sometimes, no matter what you do and how hard you try, you will not be successful. If your child had cancer and you couldn't save them, would you blame yourself? A parent can't always fix things. This doesn't mean that you give up, although some do, and for good reason.

Seven, understand that while you love a person who is ill and because of that you hurt, that person is the one with the mental illness and what they are going through can be more horrific than what most of us will ever imagine. Learn to listen, treat them with respect, try to build trust, and when possible, become a partner—make sure they are part of the solution and not seen as a problem that needs to be fixed.

What I have learned is that for me, ultimately, I must have hope. I must believe that recovery is possible. I must believe because without hope, I know recovery will never happen.

You have to believe that a better day is coming tomorrow.

## Be There for Others

Without a doubt, the number one piece of advice our activists provided is "listen."

Christinea Beane listens to people's stories and creates a unique piece of jewelry that incorporates their experiences.

Christina Wolfgram sums her advice up succinctly:

*Be kind and listen.*

Karyl Beal's quilts share the stories of people lost to suicide.

Miana Bryant's groups for college students offer support and a place to talk about their experiences without feeling stigmatized.

And Gabe Howard reminds us that it is essential to create a safe space to share our stories and listen as we do.

Thank you for caring for those with a mental health diagnosis, their families, and their caregivers.

# AFTERWORD

**Activism is a way to master something challenging and giving to others is often a positive pathway to healing.**

—DR. KEN DUCKWORTH

Becoming a mental health activist is important, as there is still so much to be done. It can also be a great gift to have a mission that you can believe in. This is an unintended and positive side effect of activism. I have myself benefited from becoming an advocate and connecting with others who have done so. I am always learning from my fellow activists. Once you take in how much shame, prejudice, and discrimination still exists in the world for people who live with mental health conditions, activism is a logical next step.

It can also be fun to make a difference.

There are activism needs for one person at a time, and activism on a bigger, macro scale. Helping a person find care and lending an ear and an open heart to a person dealing with a mental health condition are great examples of one-to-one advocacy. Opening yourself up and sharing your own experience is another. Advocating for better care of yourself is also activism.

Together we are changing minds and making it easier for people to discuss these topics. Isolation is a core problem for many and results in delays in help-seeking for some.

In this way, openness itself is a form of advocacy. Mental health and illness are becoming a *we* process instead of a *they* process and that can further motivate each of us.

Together we have made many changes for the good, but there is much to be done. On a macro level, many people have shared their stories, and focus on legislatures and media to produce activism outcomes. For example, activism has helped to enact Mental Health Parity legislation, which prohibits insurance companies from discriminating against people with mental health conditions and substance use disorders. Activism has also helped to create a national network of early psychosis programs that offer strength-based supports to young people early in their course of symptoms. These programs offer better outcomes and more support to families than traditional care. The recent *988 legislation*, which will offer an alternative to 911 police response for mental health crises, is another good example of macro change only made possible by activism. None of these changes would be possible without people who wanted to change the ways things are.

I am working on a book project, NAMI's first. *You Are Not Alone: The NAMI Guide to Mental Illness and Recovery*, will be a practical hands-on guide to support people with first person expertise and easy to follow research. I am in the process of interviewing people who want to share their story in order to help others. This too is activism. I have found that activism is a common theme in recovery for many people I have interviewed. [Editor's note: this book's co-author Trish Lockard will be featured in Ken's book.]

Like those featured in *Make a Difference with Mental Health Activism*, I have found many inspiring people who are using their own talents to serve others in this essential mission. Like the activism leaders in this book, the people I am interviewing find many ways to give to others. They may become peer specialists, form clubs at their school, use art to heal, or become NAMI resources to teach others. They might support or encourage one person or try to change their local service system or testify at congress.

Activism is a way to master something challenging and giving to others is often a positive pathway to healing. This important work is not done, and we will need more activists to help the cause.

Come join us.

*Ken Duckworth MD*

*Chief Medical Officer NAMI National*

# MENTAL HEALTH RESOURCES

## Helplines

National Suicide Prevention Lifeline: **800-273-8255**

NAMI Helpline: **800-950-6264**

The Trevor Project (LGBTQ+ youth): **866-488-7386**

Veteran's Crisis Line: **800-273-8255**

Substance Abuse and Mental Health Services National Helpline: **1-800-662-HELP** (4357)

## Organizations

**National Alliance on Mental Illness**

This grassroots organization provides resources, educational programs, and a blog.

www.NAMI.org

On Facebook at https://www.facebook.com/NAMI

On Twitter at https://twitter.com/NAMICommunicate

### Mental Health America

This organization provides resources, information, and online mental wellness tests.

MHA https://mhanational.org/

MHA Facebook https://www.facebook.com/mentalhealthamerica

MHA Twitter

https://twitter.com/MentalHealthAm

### Substance Abuse and Mental Health Services Administration

SAMHSA is an agency within the US Department of Health and Human Services [HHS].

SAMHSA is at https://www.samhsa.gov/

## Books

*Crazy–A Father's Search Through America's Mental Health Madness*, Pete Earley, Berkley; 1st edition (April 3, 2007)

*Mental Health is an Asshole and Other Observations*, Gabe Howard, DGC Press (December 3, 2018)

*You Are Not Alone*, Dr. Ken Duckworth, Zando (Coming Fall 2022)[56]

## Podcasts

*Inside Mental Health* on Psych Central, with Gabe Howard

https://psychcentral.com/blog/show

*Sobcast the Podcast,* with Christina Wolfgram

https://open.spotify.com/show/7FaUijVZTBWak9LW34e9cE

# ACKNOWLEDGMENTS

We presented a workshop on Creative Advocacy Techniques at a National Alliance for Mental Illness Convention a few years ago. Our participants loved the idea of doing activism that matched their gifts. Although fundraising, advocacy, and lobbying will always be essential activism methods for the mental health cause, our workshop participants looked for other ways to make a difference for this community.

Our participants embraced the Activism Path and helped each other come up with creative ideas for change. The passion was palpable. And out of this experience, we knew that expanding the arsenal of activism techniques would benefit both activists and those with mental health disorders and their loved ones.

Hence, the birth of *Make a Difference with Mental Health Activism.*

We've had much help along the way.

Toni Stephenson, Kathy Martin, Aleta Ledendecker, Jill England, and Pat Luna provided feedback on an earlier draft of *Make a Difference.* Their comments and questions were invaluable to improving the book. Thank you for taking the time to read the manuscript and provide us with your thoughtful feedback.

Graphic designer bittereva created our beautiful cover. We're sure it wasn't easy to work with two authors with little artistic sense, but she was patient and creative through the process.

Thank you to Pete Earley for his example of courage in the face of his son's mental health disorder. Today, Pete's son, Kevin Earley, is in recovery[57] from bipolar disorder and self-destructive psychotic behavior. Kevin has turned what seemed like an insurmountable battle against his illness into mental health activism of the highest degree—he is a rapper, songwriter, and public speaker, sharing his struggle for all to derive encouragement from.

Thank you to Dr. Ken Duckworth for his participation in this activism book. We hope that Ken's forthcoming book *You Are Not Alone: The NAMI Guide to Mental Illness and Recovery* is just the first of many books published by this country's largest grassroots mental health organization.

Finally, we want to thank our Activists in Action: Christinea Beane, Christina Wolfgram, Karyl Chastain Beal, Miana Bryant, and Gabe Howard, for their willingness to tell their stories. It isn't easy to be vulnerable about your experience with mental illness. Still, these activists understand how their stories can help others. The range of ways they make a difference for mental health activism shows the value of finding your purpose and understanding your gifts. Thank you for making the world a better place.

# Also Available

Thank you for reading *Make a Difference with Mental Health Activism.* You might also be interested in these titles:

*What's On Your Sign? How to focus your passion and change the world*

*The What's On Your Sign?* Workbook

Contact admin@LifeAtTheIntersection.com for a Teacher's Guide to *What's On Your Sign?*

Sign up for updates at https://lifeattheintersection.com/newsletter-signup/

Join the discussion in the 5-step Activism Path Facebook Group at https://www.facebook.com/5StepPath

# About the Authors

One of the best ways to support our mental health activism is to leave a review on our Amazon book page. Let others know how the book helped you get started in mental health activism.

## Trish Lockard

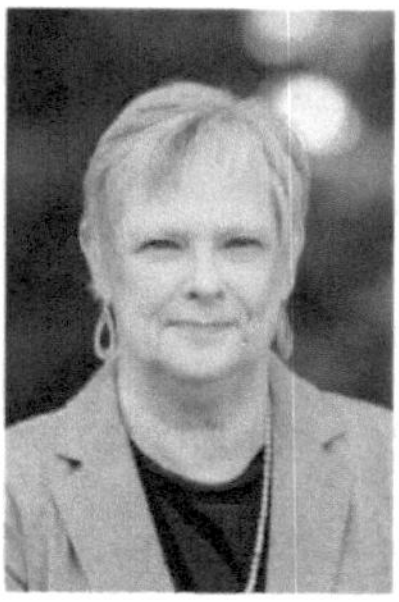

Trish Lockard is a nonfiction and creative nonfiction book editor and memoir writing coach. She freelances with publishing companies and has her own editorial services business, Strike The Write Tone.

Mental health care is a personal passion for Trish. Mental health disorders (and one incident of suicide) are a reality in four generations of her family. A long-time member of and volunteer for the National Alliance on Mental Illness (NAMI), she is a certified classroom instructor for the NAMI flagship program Family-to-Family and served several years as a local affiliate president.

Trish's Mental Health Blog Posts at Life At The Intersection:

- ✓ Think the Pandemic was Hard? Consider the Impact on Those with Mental Illness
- ✓ With Mental Illness You Won't Get a Casserole
- ✓ Stigma: A Thorn in the Side of Mental Health Care
- ✓ 12 Creative Ways to Support Mental Health

Trish's article at NAMI.org:

- ✓ Peer Support: Helping Others, Healing Yourself

To learn more about Trish:

Website: https://www.strikethewritetone.com/

Facebook: https://www.facebook.com/StrikeTheWriteTone

Twitter: https://twitter.com/WriteTone

LinkedIn: https://www.linkedin.com/in/trish-lockard-465b73159/

Instagram: https://www.instagram.com/trishlockard/

## TERRI LYON

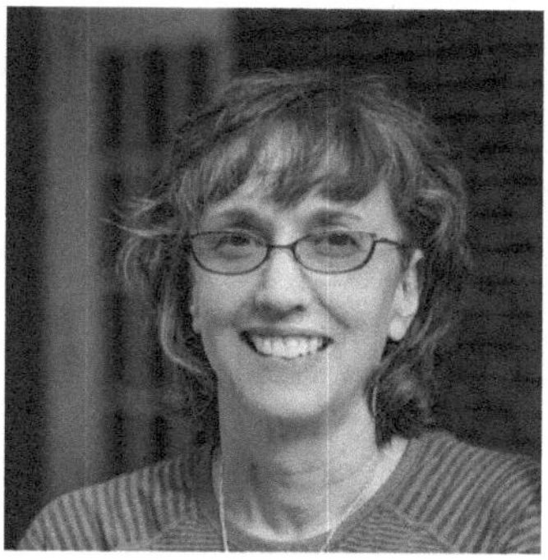

Through her website Life At The Intersection, Terri Lyon spotlights the unique, creative, and sometimes surprising ways people make change happen through their activism. A licensed psychologist, her career experience includes government research, managing training at a Fortune 500 company, consulting, and almost 40 years teaching graduate students. She is the treasurer of a credit union and a professional arbitrator for the Better Business Bureau.

To learn more about Terri and to find more resources on activism:

Read Terri's blog at https://lifeattheintersection.com/blog/

Follow Terri on Twitter @LifeAtTheIntSec

Like Terri's Facebook Page https://www.facebook.com/LifeAtTheIntSec

# Index

*Action Plan, 74*

*Activism, 13, 35, 42*

*Activism Opportunity, 81*

*Activism Techniques, 39*

*Adverse Childhood Experiences, 25*

*Advocacy, 42*

*Arts, 47*

*Caregivers, 6, 13, 24, 43*

*Celebration, 76*

*Christina Wolfgram, 29*

*Christinea Beane, 20*

*Corporate Protests, 55*

*Crafting, 48*

*Cultural Competence, 33*

*Dorothea Dix, 10*

*Dr. Ken Duckworth, 87*

*Drawing, 47*

*Fundraising, 45*

*Gabe Howard, 71*

*Gay–straight alliance, 57*

*Gifts, 29*

*Illustration, 47*

*Impact, 61, 81*

*Karyl Chastain Beal, 39*

*Kevin Earley, 2, 96*

*Knowledge, 33*

*Legal Support, 52*

*Life Vision, 23*

*Lobbying, 45*

*Logic, 49*

*Mental Health America, 91*

*Mental Health Parity and Addiction Equity Act, 8*

*Miana Bryant, 62*

*Michael Phelps, 10*

*Motivation, 34, 83*

*Movement Support, 53*

*Music, 49*

*NAMI, 3, 84, 88, 91*

*Naomi Osaka, 10*

*News Media Outreach, 52*

*Newspaper, 51*

*Parity, 8*

*Passion, 80*

*Pete Earley, 1, 84*

*Photography, 51*

*Podcasts, 54*

*Quilting, 42*

*Refocusing, 76*

*Self-Care, 75*

*Simone Biles, 10*

*Skills, 32*

*Slacktivism, 54*

*Social Media, 54*

*Stay Motivated, 71*

*Stigma, 1, 7, 11*

*Stress Awareness, 75*

*Substance Abuse and Mental Health Services Administration, 8*

*Suicide, 5, 20, 40*

*Terri Lyon, 101*

*The Activism Path, 13*

*The What's On Your Sign? Workbook, 27, 37, 58, 78*

*Theater, 48*

*Trish Lockard, 99*

*What's On Your Sign?, 27, 37, 58, 78*

*Writing, 50*

*YouTube, 54*

# Notes

We list the notes and links for *Make a Difference with Mental Health Activism* here. These are up to date as of publication, but we will keep them updated on our Mental Health Activism Companion Website.

The web address for the Mental Health Activism Companion Website is https://lifeattheintersection.com/mental-health-activism-companion/

Once you get to the Mental Health Activism Companion Website, the notes and links are organized by chapter.

If you find any mistakes, please report them to admin@lifeattheintersection.com.

## Foreword

[1] Learn more about Pete Earley's *The Hot House* at http://www.peteearley.com/books/the-hot-house/

[2] Learn more about Pete Earley's *Crazy: A Father's Search Through America's Mental Health Madness* at http://www.peteearley.com/books/crazy/

[3] The website for the National Alliance on Mental Illness (NAMI) is https://www.nami.org/

## Preface

[4] The Mental Health America quote about parity is from https://www.mhanational.org/issues/issue-brief-parity

[5] Read Trish Lockard's article on mental health during the pandemic at https://lifeattheintersection.com/2021/05/10/think-the-pandemic-was-hard-consider-the-impact-on-those-with-mental-illness

[6] Watch Lester Holt's interview with Michael Phelps (Part 1)

https://www.nbcnews.com/nightly-news/video/michael-phelps-speaks-on-importance-of-mental-health-part-1-117596229869

(Part 2) Michael Phelps Interview

https://www.nbcnews.com/nightly-news/video/michael-phelps-speaks-on-importance-of-mental-health-part-2-117594693944

[7] Learn more about Terri Lyon's *What's On Your Sign? How to focus your passion and change the world* at https://lifeattheintersection.com/

## Chapter 1

[8] Christinea Beane's Makes Cents Jewelry is at https://www.makescentsjewelry.com/

[9] Christinea Beane donates to the organization To Write Love On Her Arms. Learn more at https://twloha.com/

[10] Read more about #WearYourMeds at https://www.thelweiss.com/wear-your-meds

[11] *What's On Your Sign?* by Terri Lyon is available at Amazon.

[12] *The What's On Your Sign? Workbook* by Terri Lyon is available at Amazon.

[13] To read "How To Create A Vision of a Joyful Life" go to https://lifeattheintersection.com/2019/11/04/how-to-create-a-vision-of-a-joyful-life/

[14] To read "With Mental Illness You Won't Get A Casserole" go to https://lifeattheintersection.com/2019/05/20/with-mental-illness-you-wont-get-a-casserole/

## Chapter 2

[15] Christina's Wolfgram's Sobcast the Podcast is at https://open.spotify.com/show/7FaUijVZTBWak9LW34e9cE

[16] Mark Henson's book *Ordinary Superpowers : Unleash the Full Potential of Your Most Natural Talents* is available at Amazon.

[17] The Activist Skills and Experiences Questionnaire is at http://www.vernalproject.org/papers/change/ActQuest.pdf

[18] Take the quiz "How Privileged Are You?" at Buzzfeed https://www.buzzfeed.com/soniathomas/how-privileged-are-you

[19] At the website It's Pronounced Metrosexual you can find examples of upper-class privilege https://www.itspronouncedmetrosexual.com/2012/10/list-of-upperclass-privilege/

[20] Read "What You Can Do and What You Know Will Change The World" by Terri Lyon at https://lifeattheintersection.com/2019/08/12/what-you-can-do-and-what-you-know-will-change-the-world/

## Chapter 3

[21] View the Love Never Dies Quilts at https://tspn.org/initiatives-outreach/love-never-dies-memorial-quilt/we-remember-them/

[22] Learn more about NAMI's Family-to-Family Program https://www.nami.org/Support-Education/Mental-Health-Education/NAMI-Family-to-Family

[23] Get information about NAMI Smarts for Advocacy at https://www.nami.org/Find-Support/NAMI-Programs/NAMI-Smarts-for-Advocacy

[24] Learn about Mental Health First Aid at https://www.mentalhealthfirstaid.org/take-a-course/find-a-course/

[25] The National Suicide Prevention Hotline at https://suicidepreventionlifeline.org/our-network/

[26] Help others in distress with Question-Persuade-Refer at https://qprinstitute.com/

[27] Learn more about Make It OK https://makeitok.org/

[28] How a beer brewer makes a difference at https://www.kshb.com/news/local-news/personal-loss-prompts-lenexa-couple-to-brew-beer-for-suicide-prevention

[29] Learn more about artist Kimmy Henderson's bipolar awareness campaign at https://www.akron.com/articles/bipolar-butterfly-project-spotlights-mental-health/

[30] Learn more about Joan Baez's art at https://www.gratefulweb.com/articles/joan-baezs-mischief-makers-2-exhibition-opens-january-6

[31] The Craftivist Collective is an amazing UK resource for gentle, creative activism. https://craftivist-collective.com/

[32] Acting for the Future is theater supporting mental health. Read more at http://www.artsandhealth.ie/case-studies/acting-for-the-future/

[33] The December 2017 Vibrant.org article about rapper Logic https://www.vibrant.org/mha-nyc-logic-continue-impact/

[34] The Suicide Prevention Lifeline press release is at https://suicidepreventionlifeline.org/wp-content/uploads/2017/10/Logic-Lifeline-Press-Release-Final.pdf

[35] Learn more about Mental Health America's work at https://www.mentalhealthamerica.net/issues/advocacy-network

[36] Man Therapy Tips is at http://www.mantherapy.org/

[37] NAMI's campaigns to eliminate stigma are at https://www.nami.org/Get-Involved/Pledge-to-Be-StigmaFree/StigmaFree-Me/StigmaFree-Pledge

[38] Learn more about Big White Wall at https://www.mhinnovation.net/innovations/big-white-wall

[39] Read more about the artistic Nike shoe campaign at https://www.highsnobiety.com/p/nike-air-max-270-react-in-my-feels-release-date-price/

[40] Read "How To Find The Best Activism Method" by Terri Lyon at https://lifeattheintersection.com/how-to-find-the-best-activism-method/

## Chapter 4

[41] Miana Bryant's The Mental Elephant is at http://www.thementalelephant.com/

[42] Watch the video of Ken Duckworth and Miana Bryant on CBS Good Morning at https://www.cbsnews.com/video/how-peer-groups-like-mental-elephant-can-help-young-adults-with-mental-illness/

[43] Read "How To Make an Impact with Your Activism" by Terri Lyon at https://lifeattheintersection.com/how-to-make-impact-with-your-activism/

[44] *Doing Good Better* by William MacAskill is available at Amazon https://amazon.com/Doing-Good-Better-Effective-Altruism/dp/1592409660/ref=sr_1_1?s=books&ie=UTF8&qid=1524837589&sr=1-1&keywords=doing+good+better

## Chapter 5

[45] Gabe Howard's website https://www.gabehoward.com/

[46] The Easy Guide to the Goal Setting Process https://creately.com/blog/diagrams/goal-setting-process/

[47] Read *The Lifelong Activist* https://smile.amazon.com/Lifelong-Activist-Change-without-Losing/dp/1590560906/ref=sr_1_1?s=books&ie=UTF8&qid=1524837934&sr=1-1&keywords=the+lifelong+activist

[48] A guide for writing SMART goals at https://www.ucop.edu/local-human-resources/_files/performance-appraisal/How%20to%20write%20SMART%20Goals%20v2.pdf

[49] Learn how to deal with compassion fatigue at https://www.self.com/story/activism-fatigue

[50] A guide to gratefulness from Harvard https://www.health.harvard.edu/newsletter_article/in-praise-of-gratitude

[51] A tool for savoring happiness from Clearer Thinking http://programs.clearerthinking.org/savoring.html#.WuJifojwaUk

[52] Take a stress test from Psych Central https://psychcentral.com/quizzes/stress-test.htm

[53] Read "How To Stay Motivated In Your Activism" by Terri Lyon at https://lifeattheintersection.com/how-to-stay-motivated-in-your-activism/

## Conclusion

[54] This article about bipolar disorder contains the Demi Lovato quote mentioned here https://archive.attn.com/stories/3490/demi-lovato-bipolar-disorder

[55] Pete Earley comments that, "on average, in 2018, the cost of holding people in federal custody was $102.60 per day per adult, or $37,449 a year. The monetary cost for juvenile detention is staggering: $588 per day per youth, or $214,620 a year."

In a NAMI article, Joseph Vanable says, "The average cost for psychiatric treatment in a community hospital ranges from $3,616 to $8,509, depending on the type of illness being treated. On average, in 2018, the cost of holding people in federal custody was $102.60 per day per adult, or $37,449 a year. The monetary cost for juvenile detention is staggering: $588 per day per youth, or $214,620 a year.

The average cost for psychiatric treatment in a community hospital ranges from $3,616 to $8,509, depending on the type of illness being treated."

https://www.nami.org/Blogs/NAMI-Blog/March-2021/The-Cost-of-Criminalizing-Serious-Mental-Illness

[56] Read more about Dr. Ken Duckworth's upcoming book *You Are Not Alone*: Dr. Ken Duckworth writing mental health guide, due in 2022.

https://apnews.com/article/entertainment-coronavirus-pandemic-mental-health-b16a9032b40de3a8a9427daf9b6a1710

[57] Learn more about Kevin Earley's story at https://www.peteearley.com/2015/05/15/my-son-shares-his-recovery-story-becomes-emotional-talking-about-the-plight-of-others/

Made in United States
Troutdale, OR
11/03/2026

56845094R00076